Stories of ageing

RETHINKING AGEING SERIES

Series editor: Brian Gearing
School of Health and Social Welfare
The Open University

'Open University Press' *Rethinking Ageing* series has yet to put a foot wrong and its latest additions are well up to standard . . . The series is fast becoming an essential part of the canon. If I ever win the lottery, I shall treat myself to the full set in hardback . . .'

Nursing Times

Current and forthcoming titles:
Miriam Bernard: **Promoting health in old age**
Simon Biggs *et al.*: **Elder abuse in perspective**
Ken Blakemore and Margaret Boneham: **Age, race and ethnicity**
Joanna Bornat (ed.): **Reminiscence reviewed**
Bill Bytheway: **Ageism**
Anthony Chiva and David F. Stears (eds): **Health promotion and older people**
Maureen Crane: **Understanding older homeless people**
Mike Hepworth: **Stories of ageing**
Frances Heywood *et al.*: **Housing and home in later life**
Beverley Hughes: **Older people and community care**
Tom Kitwood: **Dementia reconsidered**
Eric Midwinter: **Pensioned off**
Sheila Peace *et al.*: **Re-evaluating residential care**
Moyra Sidell: **Health in old age**
Robert Slater: **The psychology of growing old**
John Vincent: **Politics, power and old age**
Alan Walker and Tony Maltby: **Ageing Europe**
Alan Walker and Gerhard Naegele (eds): **The politics of old age in Europe**

Stories of ageing

MIKE HEPWORTH

OPEN UNIVERSITY PRESS
Buckingham · Philadelphia

Open University Press
Celtic Court
22 Ballmoor
Buckingham
MK18 1XW

email: enquiries@openup.co.uk
world wide web: www.openup.co.uk

and
325 Chestnut Street
Philadelphia, PA 19106, USA

First Published 2000

A catalogue record of this book is available from the British Library

ISBN 0 335 19853 8 (pbk)   0 335 19854 6 (hbk)

Library of Congress Cataloging-in-Publication Data

Hepworth, Mike.
    Stories of ageing / Mike Hepworth.
      p. cm — (Rethinking ageing)
    Includes Bibliographical references and index.
    ISBN 0-335-19854-6 — ISBN 0-335-19853-8 (pbk.)
      1. English fiction—20th century—History and criticism.   2. Aging in literature.
    3. Old age in literature.   4. Aged in literature.   I. Rethinking ageing series

PR888.A394 H37 2000
823'.9109354—dc21

                                                                            00-037508

Typeset by Type Study, Scarborough
Printed in Great Britain by Biddles Limited, Guildford and Kings Lynn

Contents

Series editor's preface

As the new century begins we are some 15 books into the 'Rethinking Ageing' series. It seems appropriate therefore to review our original aims in the light of the response of readers and the concerns which gave rise to the series. The 'Rethinking Ageing' series was planned in the early 1990s, following the rapid growth in ageing populations in Britain and other countries that led to a dramatic increase in academic and professional interest in gerontology. In the 1970s and 80s there had been a steady increase in the publication of British research studies which attempted to define and describe the characteristics and needs of older people. There were also a smaller number of theoretical attempts to reconceptualize the meaning of old age and to explore new ways in which we could think about ageing. By the 1990s, however, there was a perceived gap between all that was known about ageing by gerontologists and the very limited amount of information which was readily available and accessible to the growing number of people with a professional or personal interest in old age. The 'Rethinking Ageing' series was conceived as a response to that 'knowledge gap'.

The first book to be published in the series was *Age, Race and Ethnicity* by Ken Blakemore and Margaret Boneham. In the series editor's preface we stated that the main aim of the 'Rethinking Ageing' series was to fill the knowledge gap with books which would focus on a topic of current concern or interest in ageing (ageism, elder abuse, health in later life, dementia, etc.). Each book would address two fundamental questions: What is known about this topic? And what are the policy and practice implications of this knowledge? We wanted authors to provide a readable and stimulating review of current knowledge but also to *rethink* their subject area by developing their own ideas in the light of their particular research and experience. We also believed it was essential that the books should be both scholarly and written in clear, non-technical language that would appeal equally to a broad range of students, academics and professionals with a common interest in ageing and age care.

The books published so far have ranged broadly in subject matter – from ageism to reminiscence to community care to pensions to residential care. We have been very pleased that the response from individual readers and reviewers has been extremely positive towards almost all of the titles. The success of the series appears therefore to justify its original aims. But how different is the national situation in gerontology ten years on? And do we need to adopt a different approach? The most striking change is that, today, age and ageing are prominent topics in media and government policy debates. This reflects a greater awareness in the media and amongst politicians of the demographic situation – by 2007 there will be more people over pensionable age than there will be children (*The Guardian,* 29 May 1999). However, as a recent article in *Generations Review* noted, paradoxically, the number of social gerontology courses are actually decreasing (Bernard *et al.,* Vol. 9, No. 3, September 1999). The reasons for this are not entirely clear, but they probably reflect the difficulties which today's worker-students face in securing the time and funding to attend courses. Alongside this is the pressure on course providers to respond only to the short-term training needs of care staff through short, problem-focused modules. Only a few gerontology courses are based around an in-depth and truly integrated curriculum that combines the very many different academic disciplines and professional perspectives which contribute to our knowledge and understanding of ageing.

There appears to be even more interest in ageing and old age than when we started the 'Rethinking Ageing' series, and this persuades us that there is likely to be a continuing need for the serious but accessible topic-based books in ageing that it has offered. The uncertainties about the future of gerontological education reinforce this view. However, having now addressed many of the established, mainstream topics, we feel it is time to extend its subject-matter to include 'emerging topics' and those whose importance have yet to be widely appreciated. Among the first books to reflect this policy were Maureen Crane's *Understanding Older Homeless People* and John Vincent's *Politics, Power and Old Age.* (More recently, Miriam Bernard's *Promoting Health in Old Age* combined elements of both the mainstream and the emergent.)

Mike Hepworth's *Stories of Ageing* is another groundbreaking publication. It is the first book by an author based in the UK to explore the potential of literary fiction as a gerontological resource. *Stories of Ageing* combines an approach based firmly in sociological theory with detailed analyses of many contemporary novels that deal with aspects of ageing. Drawing on his study of more than 100 works of fiction – both 'popular' and 'literary' – Hepworth's book demonstrates in fascinating detail how these can be sources of insight into the self in later life.

We believe that the publication of *Stories of Ageing* is an exciting development for the 'Rethinking Ageing' series, and one which reflects a growing interest in using humanistic and artistic sources to gain insights into old age. In future, we hope to continue to rethink ageing by revisiting topics already dealt with (via second editions of existing titles) and by finding new titles which can extend the subject matter of the series.

Brian Gearing
School of Health and Social Welfare
The Open University

Acknowledgements

Writing is an interactive process, and over several years I have learned to appreciate the creative endeavours of the novelists whose stories are cited in this book. I hope that readers who are not already familiar with their work will find these novels equally stimulating and enjoyable.

Marian, my wife, who has been unstinting in her encouragement and support, meticulously scrutinized drafts of each chapter, and the final version. Guy, my son, supplied the kind of IT support that someone who is easily frustrated by the apparently inexplicable vagaries of technology finds invaluable.

Brian Gearing was a most responsive editor, and I have benefited considerably from our conversations and his constructive comments. Jonathan Ingoldby provided just the right blend of precision and support in his professional editing of the typescript which an author requires when the end of the road appears to be in sight.

Introduction

This book is about stories of ageing. By stories of ageing I mean full-length novels which are about ageing as experienced by a central character or a small group of characters such as a married couple or a family. Under this heading I also include stories where ageing may not be the main interest of the writer but which include significant references to aspects of the ageing process or to older people. A large number of short stories about ageing have been written but with the exception of excerpts from the popular stories of James Herriot (*If Only They Could Talk* and *All Things Wise and Wonderful*), and those of David Renwick, the author of the widely acclaimed TV situation comedy on ageing, *One Foot in The Grave*, these are not included in this book. The reason is not because short stories are irrelevant – quite the contrary – but simply lack of space. My main aim in writing this book is to encourage you as readers to explore fiction as an imaginative resource for understanding variations in the meaning of the experience of ageing in society and to go out and make your own selection from the increasingly wide range of novels available. If you do so then this book will have been a success.

By 'ageing' I mean the period usually described as the later part of life; that is, the period in the life course following on from the years normally labelled '50+'. But I do not treat this label as anything more than a social convenience; following mainstream gerontological thinking I treat ageing not simply as a matter of chronology or biology but as a complex and potentially open-ended process of interaction between the body, self and society. Ageing, as gerontological research shows, is not a straightforward linear trajectory towards inevitable physical, personal and social decline but a dynamic process of highly variable change: ageing is simultaneously a collective human condition and an individualized subjective experience. To borrow a neat phrase from the novelist Reginald Hill, 'up and down like a fiddler's elbow' (1999: 311).

In social gerontology the term 'life course' is normally preferred in direct contrast with the concept of the 'life cycle' as a relatively fixed series of biologically determined stages through which natural life-forms move. The use of the sociological term 'course' indicates the comparative open-endedness of the 'stages', 'phases' or 'periods' into which human life is conventionally divided (Cohen 1987). In other words, the life 'cycle' of the fruit fly is determined by natural processes over which the fly has no conscious control, whereas the 'stages' or 'periods' of the human life course are not exclusively determined by biology but constructed by human beings and therefore, potentially at least, are open to individual and collective control.

In the chronological scale indicated by the symbol '50+' the point where individuals and groups begin to 'grow older' or 'enter' old age is not universally fixed for all time but historically and culturally variable (Gullette 1997). The social construction of the age of retirement at 60/65 is a good historical example. For this reason I have a preference for the term 'ageing *into* old age'. Ageing into old age is a constant reminder that during the years '50+' the point of entry into old age is literally, as I have already noted, a symbolic construct which is interactively produced as individuals attempt to make sense of the later part of life. Individuals 'enter into' old age at different points during the life course. In this looser definition of ageing, the constitutive strands of the process – biological (body); psychological (self); and society (culture and social structure) – are not seen as distinctive factors which can be separated out but as woven closely together into the fabric of everyday social life. As the sociologist Norbert Elias (1985) has shown, our biological lives are so closely integrated with culture and the configurations of interdependencies that make up our social relationships that it is impossible to disentangle them. We are at once individuals and collective social beings. In this book, therefore, the word 'ageing' should be read throughout as shorthand for 'ageing into old age'. And I write with two assumptions.

First, that ageing is never simply a fixed biological or chronological process, but an open-ended subjective and social experience. The subjective experience of one's own ageing is potentially highly variable depending on the meanings given to the body and the self. Second, that ageing should always be understood in terms of a tension between subjective experience and the human fate we all share of a limited life span. For, as Kathleen Woodward has observed, ageing 'necessarily cuts across all our lives and our bodies in a way that other differences fundamentally do not' (1991: 156). In other words, as my father was fond of reminding me, old age 'comes to us all'. But the good news is that this shared predicament gives all of us 'a stake in representations of old age and the ageing body' (Woodward 1991: 156) and it is with this stake that this book is primarily concerned.

In making my selection from the wide range of novels available I have chosen stories which I hope for the most part are more likely to be familiar to readers. Gerontologists with an interest in fiction increasingly regard novels as an important source of information about the meanings of ageing (Bytheway 1995) and readers will probably have read at least a few of the stories cited in this book and will almost certainly have heard of several of the titles. Some are popular in the sense of being bestsellers and, following the trend of media interest in ageing, a number have either been made into films or transmitted as adaptations for television. (Examples include novels as diverse as Kingsley Amis' *Ending Up*, Nina Bawden's *Family Money*, Laurie Lee's *Cider With Rosie*, Ruth Rendell's *Simisola*, Vita Sackville-West's *All Passion Spent*, and Minette Walters' *The Scold's Bridle*). In addition, I also make occasional references to book versions of the popular television series *Last of the Summer Wine* (Roy Clarke's *Gala Week*), and David Renwick's previously mentioned collection of short stories from his TV series *One Foot in The Grave*. Hopefully the familiarity of many of these stories will make it possible for readers to compare my interpretation with their own and those of friends and colleagues, thus facilitating a more active interaction between reader and text than perhaps is possible in the academic literature on ageing.

Old age has been described as the ultimate challenge for the novelist because it is about people who are living through the final period of their lives; a time when those who live long enough have to come to terms with changes in their bodies and the attitudes of society to growing older. Stories of ageing are faced with the problem of describing a character and his or her relationships with other people when she or he has apparently little distance left to travel in the 'journey of life'. In western culture this period has usually been regarded as one of decline; a time of gradual disengagement from worldly activities when the consolations of religion are the main resource for making sense of ageing and drawing comfort from the belief that the physical decrepitude normally associated with old age is a tiresome prelude to the liberation of the essential self (soul) from the flesh into eternal life (Cole 1992). But more recently, as life expectancy for the majority has increased, people are looking for ways of replacing or extending this scenario and finding new images of positive meaning to life after 50 (Hockey and James 1993; Gullette 1997; Hepworth 1999).

In this context my purpose in writing this book is not to offer a final definitive analysis of images of ageing in fiction (even if this were remotely possible) but to encourage readers to make their own selection of stories of ageing and to look for additional or alternative interpretations of growing older to the ones I have made. The whole point, as Gullette (1988, 1993, 1997) has vividly shown in her analyses of fictional representations of ageing, is to discover how our personal ideas about ageing (positive/negative/ambiguous) are shaped by our culture and are therefore open to the possibility of change.

For ours is probably the most age-conscious period in human history. Everyday experience and the findings of gerontological research repeatedly confirm our fascination with images of ageing into old age (Featherstone and Hepworth 1993). And over the last 20 years or so the value of fictional representations of ageing has been recognized in a number of ways.

First, gerontologists occasionally draw on fiction to illustrate the findings of empirical research or to interweave gerontology and fiction in order to enhance our understanding of ageing. Valuable examples can be found in Johnson and Slater's reader, *Ageing and Later Life* (1993).

Second, there are a number of compilations of wide-ranging extracts from fiction (including poetry) where fiction is sampled to illustrate the ageing process. These texts often present a humanistic perspective on ageing within the traditional framework of the life course as a series of 'ages' and 'stages' from the cradle to the grave. They are usually a celebration of the richness and diversity of literary images of ageing, a good example being *The Oxford Book of Ageing: Reflections on the Journey of Life*, edited by Cole and Winkler (1994).

Third, there is the emergence, particularly in the USA, of 'literary gerontology' where experts in literary criticism and the history of literature have drawn on gerontological research (often from a psychological/developmental perspective) to carry out in-depth analysis of particular texts or writers. Examples include Anne Wyatt-Brown's study of the influence on the later novels of the English writer Barbara Pym of her own experiences of ageing and terminal illness:

> Her final work, *A Few Green Leaves*, returns to the village setting of her first novel. Yet Pym's life had changed too radically simply to revert to the style of her youth, for not only had she become famous, but she discovered she was dying of cancer. . . . Therefore she added a new note: the mature acceptance of death as part of the life cycle.
>
> (Wyatt-Brown 1988: 837)

Wyatt-Brown shows how ageing and the onset of cancer added a new dimension to Pym's work as she came to terms with her own mortality. *A Few Green Leaves* was published in 1980 and her previous novel, the bleaker *Quartet in Autumn* was concerned with the problems of retirement facing four older people who had worked together in the same office: Letty, Marcia, Norman and Edwin. The central theme, as Wyatt-Brown notes, is 'retirement . . . viewed quite differently by retirees and observers' (1992: 124). *Quartet in Autumn* was written at a time when Pym was becoming increasingly aware of growing older and facing the problem of assessing her future.

There are, therefore, signs of an increasing gerontological appreciation of the value stories of ageing can add to our understanding of the subtleties of the subjective experience of ageing (Zeilig 1997). And Wyatt-Brown has given one significant reason for this emerging interest – namely the contribution writing and reading stories can make to the issue of making sense of the differences between the perspectives of insiders and outsiders on ageing and death. Fiction is a particularly valuable resource precisely because it allows the writer, through the exercise of imagination, access to the personal variations and ambiguities underlying the common condition of growing older. An 84-year-old schoolmaster interviewed by Ronald Blythe for his now classic *The View in Winter*, said old age 'doesn't necessarily mean that one is entirely old – *all* old . . . which is why it is so very difficult. It is complicated by the retention of a lot of one's youth in an old body. I tend to look upon other old men as *old men* – and not include myself' (1981: 226) The idea that ageing is not a uniform process which completely eliminates the past self – 'the retention of a lot of one's youth' – points to the essential individuality of the experience of old age as a kind of mask. Writing within the academic context of sociological theorizing, Katz (1996: 1) made a related point when he observed that no 'single knowledge' of ageing is possible because the 'meanings of ageing and old age are scattered, plural, contradictory, and enigmatic. . . . Age is everywhere, but the world's cultures have taught us that age has no fixed locus'.

These quotations from Blythe and from Katz show how the diverse meanings of ageing coexist at both individual and cultural levels. Ageing exists in the mind of Blythe's schoolmaster in the form of a conscious reflection on personal ideas and beliefs about his changing body and self as he remembers it in the past. His experience of ageing is in effect an act of comparison between his subjective vision of himself as an older individual and the appearance of the other older people he is in a position to observe. His observations make a connective link with Katz's reference to the role of the wider symbolic world of culture. There is here an interactional process which in certain respects is comparable with the individual experience of reading a story of ageing; a comparison which immediately raises questions concerning the relationship between the author, the text and the reader. As the work of literary gerontologists clearly shows (see, for example, Gullette 1988, 1993; Wyatt-Brown 1988, 1992), evidence about the aims and intentions of creative writers when they address issues of ageing is difficult to unearth and dangerous to interpret. Quite simply, writers vary in the use they make of ageing as a subject for a story – there are significant differences between the in-depth analyses of the ageing self found in, for example, Pat Barker, Penelope Lively, Julian Rathbone, and May Sarton, the tragi-comedy of ageing in the work of David Renwick, and the manipulation of popular stereotypes of ageing found in some of the work of crime novelist Agatha Christie. Huge difficulties also stand in the way of making accurate assessments of the use readers make of texts. The experience of reading stories – the sense you or I make of, say, Nina Bawden's *Family Money* – may well vary widely because reading is simultaneously a private act and a social act. Reading is a process of symbolic interaction where the reader has some freedom to interpret the text according to his or her own ideas, emotions and consciousness of self. Because reading is the exercise of a social skill engaging the private self it is dangerous to make assumptions about how other people interpret the stories of ageing they read.

And yet amidst all these problems of interpretation one thing is abundantly clear. Fiction evidently adds a further dimension to our understanding of the quality of the ageing experience. Because fiction is a creative mental activity requiring author and reader to extend her or himself imaginatively into the minds of other characters, novels are in the advantageous position of admitting readers to a variety of different perspectives on the situation of an ageing individual – the view of grandma's ageing, for example, from the positions of different members of her family in Margaret Forster's *Have the Men Had Enough?* This space, opened up by creative licence, enhances the reader's appreciation of the subjective experiences of someone who is consciously aware of the process of growing older. A sense of sadness, for example, one of the emotions often associated with ageing, is movingly described in the following extract from Celia Dale's crime story with the ironic title *A Helping Hand*. The subject is Mrs Fingal, a wealthy, lonely, widow befriended by a middle-aged couple, Josh and Maisie Evans. Even when seated comfortably in their garden (they have taken her into their home):

> Sad thoughts came to her when her bones ached, although she concealed this too; thoughts all of the past, happiness taken away, loved ones who had died but who still peopled her head and her heart, so vigorous, so alive in her recollection that they forced themselves out of her mouth, a stream, a dream of what she had been when life was still happening to her. She tried to dress her memories gaily, for she was aware that even people as kind as Mr Evans were embarrassed by sadness. . . .
>
> (Dale 1990b: 60)

In this book I make no claim to offer a definitive or final analysis of an author's motivation, the content of a text or the reader's interpretation (even supposing for one moment that this would be possible). My interest is basically in the *potential* of fictional representations of ageing to engage our interest and concern. Undoubtedly the emotions, long neglected in studies of ageing, are engaged by certain stories (Hepworth 1998). Ultimately, writing and reading are processes of emotional and intellectual interaction where symbols – words – are the currency. As readers we interact with the text in terms of our understanding of the words before us; and this understanding involves an interplay between shared meanings (for example, of words such as 'ageing'; 'old'; 'declining years'; 'later life') and our own personalized versions of them ('my' ageing; my 'old age'; 'my' declining years; 'my' later life, as distinct from yours or the ageing of the characters in a novel).

In this book I have attempted to interpret my selection of stories of ageing within a 'symbolic interactionist' framework. Symbolic interactionism is one of the branches of sociology that places a high value on the role of the imagination in the development of the concept of the self. According to symbolic interactionism our sense of individual selfhood develops from infancy through the human capacity to become aware of the way others see us. An awareness of personal selfhood depends on the human ability to imagine the perspective of the other: to put ourselves, in other words, into other people's shoes. The self is not seen as something we are born with but as emerging out of interaction with other human beings and continually shaped by interaction with other people throughout the entire life course. The self, then, is a kind of social gift reflecting the essential interdependency of every one of us.

One significant aspect of our interdependency is our reliance on shared meanings in order to communicate with each other. If our ability to reciprocate is in some way impaired, the resulting breakdown in communications can produce interpersonal difficulties as the following example from Marika Cobbold's *Guppies For Tea* shows. Here Amelia is discussing the difficulties of looking after her beloved grandmother Selma who is an invalid and becoming confused:

> 'That's what's so disconcerting.' Amelia stirred the earthenware pan filled with vegetable soup. 'One moment she's the old Selma; with it, sensible, the sort of person you feel you can go to with your problems. Next thing you know, whoosh, she's gone, replaced by this large, malfunctioning child.' She looked across the kitchen at Gerald. 'It's really very upsetting.'
>
> (Cobbold 1993: 47)

It is unlikely that everyone who has just read this passage will have also read the novel from which it was taken, but few, I imagine, will have any problems understanding the meaning of the words. The shared meaning seems very clear but the personal implications for each one of us who reads this passage may well be very different, depending on our own experience and observations of dementia and infantilization, which is the process through which we perceive old age as a reversion to a 'second childhood' of dependency on others.

Ageing is at once collective and personal (the population of the world is ageing/I am ageing; but the two are not the same though they may well coincide at certain salient points). My gerontology students often include in their essays the phrase 'ageing is very much a personal and individual experience' and it is not unusual for academic writers on the social dimensions of ageing to include some reference to their personal interest and motives. In his carefully researched socio-economic history of middle age in twentieth-century Britain, John Benson refers to his own experience of ageing into middle age:

> I know a good deal about middle age. I started this book when I was 48, and finished it when I was 51. When I was 48 I celebrated my silver wedding anniversary, when I was 49 I was told that I might have glaucoma, when I was 50 I received birthday cards saying that although I didn't look fifty I probably had done once, and when I was 51 my wife and I decided to save seriously for retirement.
>
> (Benson 1997: viii)

T.R. Cole's *The Journey of Life*, a vivid and painstakingly researched history of ageing in American culture, opens with memories of his family and his grandparents and the explicit acknowledgement of his 'search for personal meaning' (1992: xvii) in ageing as a motive for his investigation of changing attitudes and perceptions. In quite a different kind of book, Kathleen Woodward's sophisticated literary and psychoanalytic analysis of ageing and poetry writing *at last, The Real Distinguished Thing* (1980), there is a reference in the preface to her personal reasons for her academic interest in the later work of poets such as T.S. Eliot, Ezra Pound and Wallace Stevens. Woodward's second book, *Ageing and Its Discontents* (1991) is the result, she confesses, of a painful personal awareness as a younger person of the physical difficulties experienced by older relatives – what she calls the 'darker tone' of her work (1991: 23). Here she concentrates more closely on the contribution of imaginative fiction to our understanding of the limitations of our biologically ageing bodies. The book contains a number of painful recollections of much-loved relatives in old age, describing, for example, the last days of her grandmother in the hospital wing of a retirement home:

> My grandmother had been there for years. She was all bones, curled up into herself. She muttered and murmured to herself. I could not make out what she was saying. I wanted to know what she was thinking, what she was feeling. She had never cultivated a language of intimacy, or at least not to my knowledge. Now she was physically incapable of communicating her experience. And I did not have the resources to imagine

her experience. It seemed to me at that infinitely expandable moment that youth and age were indeed the greatest opposites of which life is capable, as Freud had remarked. I wanted a sense of her subjectivity, which so definitively escaped me. Hence, perhaps, this book. I wish too that the endings of the lives of my other grandparents, so painfully stretched out in incapacity, had been different and their experience more accessible to me. And hence, perhaps, my emphasis on the discontents of ageing.

(Woodward 1991: 24–5)

It is worthwhile comparing the above autobiographical quotation with the excerpt from Marika Cobbold's fictionalized description of infantilization previously cited. Again, readers will have no problem in understanding the dilemma expressed in Woodward's poignant account though, again, different readers will doubtless react in different ways. Reference to the personal nature of our interest in ageing inevitably raises the issue of identification; that is, the identification of the reader with characters in a novel, with the story-line, or with certain of the main themes. In *Safe at Last in the Middle Years,* Margaret Gullette has defined identification as 'the fundamental *condition of possibility*' (1988: xvi). By 'possibility' she means not only the resource provided by the entire range of stories of ageing that are actually written down and published, but the wider freedom we enjoy to make our own interpretations of these stories and our ability to creatively develop and expand their themes. We are not, therefore, merely passive readers of fictional representations of ageing but actively engaged in using these books to make sense of our own experience of growing older. In her study of creativity, ageing and gender, Gullette (1993) argues that a critically engaged reading of fiction invites readers to explore the possibility of alternative images of ageing; to 'think age' in a new and positive way. Her view is that a critical attitude towards stories of ageing sharpens our awareness of the tension between the shared vocabularies of ageing and our personal experience and expectations: 'once we begin to think age, a more mysterious and intangible project emerges: to discover what our own culture is serving up for us, and what each of us has consumed or resisted' (Gullette 1993: 46).

Stories of Ageing should be read in the light of Gullette's critical perspective. As the products of historically established systems of ideas and beliefs about ageing stories make a significant contribution to 'thinking age'. Novels are one source of our ideas and beliefs about ageing which, to borrow again from Gullette, offer 'material for the use of different readers', and readers will 'take what they can use' from the book (Gullette 1988: 45).

Stories of Ageing is an invitation to explore fiction as one source of ideas about the ageing process and their possible influence over our individual subjective experience of growing older in contemporary society. It should be read as an exploration of fictional images of ageing in a selection of novels published during the period from the 1930s to the present day. All the novels cited are fully referenced under the heading 'Fiction' at the end of the book but readers should note that the date of publication is the date of the copy I have consulted and not necessarily the date when the book was first published. It is not a chronological history of themes of ageing in fiction, but is intended to be an exploration of one of the key issues involved in an understanding of the experience of ageing – namely processes of interaction between the body, self and other people. The key issues of ageing in Chapters 2 to 6 – body and self; self and others; objects, places and spaces; vulnerability and risk; and futures – can be cross-referenced with mainstream questions concerning biological ageing, the ageing self, friendship, dependency, loneliness, caring, the emotions, the quality of life, successful and unsuccessful ageing, and the future of ageing found in most gerontological textbooks (see Bond *et al.* 1993). The main difference between this book and other texts in social gerontology is the use of examples drawn from the world of the creative imagination, as seen from a symbolic interactionist perspective.

While the novels I have chosen focus on particular aspects of the ageing experience, I suggest that they can be linked via the insights of symbolic interactionism with more general or universal ideas about ageing as a process which has emerged from gerontological research over the last few decades. Diane Vaughan has noted that the key problem in sociology is the tension between the individual and society. Sociology, she argues, is 'only possible because human behaviour is patterned' but at the same time 'the path of each individual life is unique and unpredictable' (1988: 9). The same difficulty, as I noted above, pervades discussions of understanding ageing, and the structure of the book – the particular framing of stories of ageing – sets out to reflect the interplay between the body, the self and society in the six chapters.

The chapter headings indicate key aspects of the ageing process as analysed from a symbolic interactionist perspective. Chapter 1 introduces the symbolic interactionist approach in greater detail and highlights areas of correspondence between symbolic interactionism and stories as meaningful narratives of ageing. I also provisionally distinguish five variations in the themes of stories of ageing in terms of the quality, depth and intensity of focus on key aspects of ageing as an interactive process.

In Chapter 2 I take a closer look at the interaction between the body and the self, taking the view that although ageing is ultimately grounded or 'embodied' in biological change – if the body did not age there would literally be no gerontological story to write or read – the relationship between body and self raises important questions about the meaning of the life course with which we have to struggle as we grow older.

Chapter 3 develops this interactional theme further, to expand on the role of relationships between the body, the self and other people. In Chapter 4 I extend the interactional chain to include the interdependency of self on objects (the symbolic role of 'biographical objects', Hoskins 1998, in shaping the self) and the part played by places and spaces (such as the 'home' and the residential 'home') in shaping age identities.

One of the central issues in any discussion of ageing is the problem of the specific risks associated with physical frailty and with particular places and spaces, such as a high crime area of an inner city, and Chapter 5 looks at examples of the dangers to which older people are exposed. I also extend the concept of risk to include what in one sense may be interpreted to be more positive aspects of risk – as displayed in fictional treatments of older people as risk *takers* – and sometimes as posing a threat to other (including younger) people. Finally in Chapter 6 I take up the question of the future of human ageing in relation to the interplay between past, present and future in the life course.

Because ageing is ultimately about human constructs of the meanings of life and time these ideas inevitably exercise a significant influence over the ways in which we make sense of growing older. Much of our thinking about later life takes place within a framework of the 'ages' and 'stages of life' inherited from past times, which are in certain respects very different from our own (Cole 1992). It may well be that the models of the life course we have inherited will be much less appropriate in years to come – the 'decline narrative' in fiction has recently come under sustained critical attack (Gullette 1988, 1993, 1997) – but there is a still a long way to go and the future largely remains, as it has always been, a matter of speculation.

1

Stories of ageing

The main theme of this book is the contribution fictional descriptions of ageing can make to our understanding of ageing as a socio-psychological process. Stories of ageing are regarded as a cultural resource each individual can draw upon to enhance his or her appreciation of the subjective and inter-personal dimensions of the experience of ageing. As previously indicated, the main conceptual framework of this book is sociological, and the stories I have selected to write this particular story of ageing have been interpreted from a symbolic interactionist perspective.

This chapter has three aims. First, to introduce the key ideas of symbolic interactionism. Second, to review the symbolic interactionist perspective on stories as narratives. And third, to describe five variations in the stories of ageing which I have selected for this book.

Symbolic interactionism

Symbolic interactionism is an attractive conceptual framework for under-standing the experience of ageing for two basic reasons, one following from the other. Namely, the central role symbols and images play in the social organization of human life and consequently the central role played by symbols in the creation of the individual human self.

To put the whole issue into a nutshell, human life is not instinctual but social, and as such it has a long history (Elias 1985). Because human beings are essentially interdependent creatures, relying on each other for survival and support, life is fundamentally a socially organized cooperative activity. Unlike animals whose behaviour is largely determined by inherited instinc-tual patterns of motivation, human life derives motivation and meaning from the social and cultural context. That is to say, it requires the ability to co-operate and communicate in situations where individuals meet and interact according to certain rules and expectations. The basis of cooperative activity is communication, and the characteristic feature of human communication is the symbol. We relate to each other not in terms of basic instinctual drives but through complex patterns of symbols indicated by words like 'mother', 'father', 'brother', 'friend', 'enemy', 'youth', 'middle age', 'ageing', 'old age', 'grannie', 'grandfather', 'incontinence', 'care assistant', 'matron', 'director of human resources', and so on. Without our inherited cultural repertoire of symbols, human life would not be possible. A good test of the key role of symbols in everyday life is to try to live without them. (In fact one of the problems of later life is the risk of losing the capacity to communicate symbolically through failure to recognize or remember the images that connect each individual self with others – diaries, photographs, newspapers, material possessions, places and stories about the self are the connective tissue of social life).

Symbols, comprising visual and verbal images, are an essential feature of human interaction and communication (i.e. the 'interaction' that is 'symbolic'). It is symbols that transform higher-order animals into human beings, enabling us to move beyond the basic biological conditions of our existence to experience a sense of personal identity or selfhood in the world of ideas and the imagination. According to Norbert Elias, it is symbols which free human beings from innate or instinctual patterns of behaviour; a process he describes as 'symbol emancipation' liberating us 'from the bondage of largely unlearned or innate signals and [leading to] the transition to the dominance of largely learned patterning of one's voice for the purposes of communication' (1991: 53). As the cultural heritage of our long-term cultural history, symbols extend the human imagination and potential and open up the prospect of future change.

Social interaction is therefore accomplished through the symbolic communication of shared meanings. As Gubrium has observed in his study of Alzheimer's sufferers and their carers in the USA, personal troubles like senile dementia have to be expressed in a language which is shared. In his sociological analysis the problem of Alzheimer's disease is constructed and communicated in symbolic terms when it is described variously as ' "a funeral that never ends" ', a disease that ' "makes shells of former selves" ', or metaphorically as a thief who ' "steals the mind" ' (Gubrium 1986: 119). These emotive symbols are the 'public cultures' through which private troubles are expressed and one carer relates meaningfully to another (Gubrium 1986: 118). Our understanding of ageing, therefore, is formed and given structure through the symbols we use to make sense of this ambiguous complex of biological, psychological and social changes. One set of images Gubrium chooses to illustrate his analysis of the role of symbols in giving meaning to Alzheimer's disease is the poetry composed by caregivers and sometimes sufferers themselves. These poems are again highly emotive, putting into words the subjective feelings aroused by an awareness of memory loss in the 'victims' themselves and the sadness and despair experienced by carers watching the decline in the 'mental life' of a loved one (Gubrium 1986: 128). They provide, in Gubrium's words, 'insight into the link between privacy and culture.' (1986: 128). Here is one example:

On one occasion, in a support group, a caregiving wife, who, having presented her feelings, paused for a moment, fetched a piece of paper from
her purse, and remarked, 'I clipped this out of a paper and I just wanted
to read it to you because – it's a poem – it puts into words what I think
we all feel but find it hard to communicate.' She then read the poem. In
her audience's focused attention and responses afterward, it was evident
that these special words somehow penetrated and conveyed the com-
monality of their sentiments, the 'thing' they all shared but couldn't
describe, something now being collectively represented and communicated. In the poem, they unified their distressing privacies and, as such,
recognised the depth of their common experience. As someone quietly
responded, 'That says it all.'

(Gubrium 1986: 128)

Poetry, of course, is one form of storytelling. As recorded in Gubrium's
research it is a cultural resource carers draw on to create a sense of social solidarity – they are all facing a common experience – and also to give meaning
to the ageing experiences of those they care for and to symbolically prolong
the continuity of their personal identity. In this sense poetry is a medium for
constructing both the self of the 'victim' and of her or his carer.

The social and personal significance of the role of storytelling in making
sense of ageing is also confirmed by Dorothy Jerrome in her research into old
people's clubs on the south coast of England. Stories are not only read in
privacy but are publications which are exchanged between individuals to
cement group solidarity. Jerrome describes how a set of library books published by the magazine *Woman's Weekly* was used to maintain contact between
a group of older women and one member who seemed to be in danger of
losing touch with the others. Books and magazines are not only collections
of words with shared meanings but are material articles for sustaining social
relationships: 'the lending and borrowing of books and magazines is a vital
part of the club communication system' (Jerrome 1992: 40)

Symbolically created meanings are a vitally important constituent of personal and social life and are inevitably therefore a valuable source of information about the ways in which we make sense of growing older. If, for
example, we want to understand why a particular older person is dissatisfied
with his or her transfer into residential accommodation it is probably a good
idea to find out what she or he means by the word 'home' and the personal
meaning of the transition from 'home' to 'a home' (Fairhurst 1999). Similarly, the physical distress associated with illness in later life is communicated
to others symbolically in words such as 'where do you feel the pain, mother?'
– 'Down my arm, dear'. As we shall see in Chapter 2, the experience of the
ageing human body is mediated through symbolic interaction and thus
extended well beyond the flesh and blood that is the basis of our existence.

If all aspects of human life are made meaningful through the display, struc-
turing and communication of symbols – bodies, food, clothing, shelter, emotions, sexuality, childrearing, ageing and the life course – the individual
self-consciousness of each one of us can be seen as a symbolic experience.
And our sense of individuation, of being conscious of a separate identity from

the other people around us, is expressed in relational terms. That is to say, in terms of an interdependent relationship between self and others. As we shall see in more detail in Chapter 2, the self can be divided into two parts: the self privately experienced in our inner subjective world, and the self communicated to others through our interaction with the external social world. One of the problems we face throughout our lives is that these two aspects of experience are not always harmoniously integrated. Doris Lessing's *Love Again* explores the emotional vicissitudes of Sarah Durham, a woman in her sixties who self-consciously examines her emotions, her motives and the quality of her relationships when she falls in love with younger men. One of her main concerns is the propriety of love in later life. Is it appropriate for a woman aged 65 to fall in love with younger men? How does it look to others? How do these men see Sarah? What does the relationship mean to them? How does she feel about herself?

> it was not possible she was in love with a handsome youth she had nothing at all in common with except the instant sympathy she owed to his love for his mother. Perhaps when he was seventy, well pickled by life, they might mean the same thing when they used words – yes, possibly then, but she would be dead.
>
> (Lessing 1996: 104)

Love Again explores the interaction between the subjective and social dimensions of Sarah Durham's self as seen through her own eyes. Because it is about the problem of love between an older woman and younger men it highlights some of the subtleties of interpersonal interaction and the difficulties Sarah experiences in communicating her personal feelings in a society where such relationships tend to be disapproved of. The intensity of the emotions Sarah experiences and her desire to embrace them does not totally obscure her awareness of conventional attitudes towards the public expression of such desires. She is simultaneously her own person and the creature of her times, and her thought processes are a reflection of these tensions and the problems she faces in resolving them. Lessing, the novelist, uses her creative imagination to open up an aspect of the experience of ageing which is often a closely guarded personal secret – 'locked in the heart' as we sometimes say – and is certainly difficult to express in conventional words.

The symbolic meanings of the private and public self, and the tensions existing between them, have profound implications for the experience of ageing. This is because close relationships with others, like love and friendship, are only fully brought to life when a shared understanding has been established. But the achievement of such a shared understanding is itself a precarious business. Sarah Durham has to come to terms first of all with the realization that she has fallen in love with Bill and then with the problem of publicly expressing her love. As we have seen, some of her difficulties are derived from the social expectation that older women are not supposed to fall in love with younger men, and if they do they are certainly not expected to express their feelings.

It is possible to extend the interactional problem of a tension between the subjective and the social self further to include the barriers to communication that stand in the way of self-expression in later life when individuals become confused or dementing. If, for example, I begin to experience any of the problems associated with dementia – difficulty remembering the time, the day, the place, whether I have read the newspaper or not, difficulties over identifying myself in the mirror – then the relationship between myself and others may well become more and more strained as time goes on. If for some reason you don't understand what I, as an older person, am saying – if I am using what you consider to be an inappropriate language, or if I am inarticulate, confused, or have lost my memory of experiences we have shared – then I shall have problems in expressing myself to you and you may well begin to think that I am no longer my 'old self'. If for any reason my command of the symbolic resources required to express the self you recognize has been changed in some way (as happens when Sarah Durham falls in love) or seriously impaired, then in your eyes I shall cease to be my 'old' self.

A neat reference to the sequence of symbolic interpretations involved in the interplay in later life between a 'young' and an 'old' self occurs in a conversation in Reginald Hill's crime story *Exit Lines*. Here the mother-in-law of Pascoe the police detective is describing her experience of her husband's ageing:

> Pascoe looked at her thoughtfully and said, 'How long's Archie been like this, Madge?'
> 'Oh a long time,' she said vaguely. 'It's getting worse slowly, and it won't get better. But it's funny what you get used to, isn't it? And most of the time, he's still his old self. Well, that's what he is, isn't it? His *old* self. Himself, but old, I mean.'
>
> (Hill 1987: 246–7)

A number of issues are of interest here. First, Archie's growing 'worse' is a gradual and fluctuating process. Most of the time Madge perceives him as 'still his old self' yet at the same time the 'old self' is not really the self to which she has become accustomed or even a complete reversion to some younger self in the past. It is a self of old age, or what we sometimes describe as a self 'in' old age. More generally, it is important to note that these permutations of selfhood are only possible because of our sophisticated linguistic resources. Archie's self (or selves) are created and interpreted in symbolic terms. I shall return to a more detailed discussion of the symbolic interactionist analysis of the relationship between the body and the self in Chapter 2.

In the textbook *Ageing in Society*, Bond *et al.* (1993) provide a helpful overview of the contribution of symbolic interactionism to gerontology and this may be briefly summarized as follows:

• Individual and group human action is motivated by meanings.
• Language is an important symbolic resource for creating and communicating personal and social meaning.
• If we wish to understand the experience of ageing we have to understand both the personal and social meanings that individuals give to ageing – to see the world through their eyes and how they define a particular situation.
• But we also have to understand how individual older persons interact

with others. Any given situation can be described in terms of two perspectives: that of each of the individuals involved and the group perspective.

• If effective cooperative action is to be achieved, personal subjective meanings have to be communicated to other people in terms of meanings they understand. The meaning is then no longer one-sided but shared. If meanings cannot be shared with others then communication will break down or at least face the risk of being misunderstood.

If the processes of interpersonal communication break down for any reason then the individual sense of selfhood can be seriously threatened, an outcome that has been dealt with imaginatively in a number of stories of ageing. I am thinking particularly of novels where confusion and loss of memory are described subjectively through the eyes of the person with dementia, in contrast to the external perceptions of family members (usually younger) who are closely involved in the situation. Because of the variety of perspectives which are possible in imaginative fiction the reader may be guided towards a deeper understanding of the person with dementia than is available to the other main characters who are often in the role of carers.

Two examples, to which I shall return in greater detail in subsequent chapters, are Francis Hegarty's *Let's Dance* and Thea Astley's *Coda*. The central characters in these stories are women who are becoming seriously confused. Although the plots (and probably the intentions of the authors) are very different, both these stories are novels with the subjective experience of confusion as a core theme. *Coda* opens with Kathleen's admission that she is losing control over her memories and that her subjective experience of herself is changing: 'she was starting to think of herself in the third person' (Astley 1995: 5). It unfolds as a confused medley of Kathleen's memories of the past, and her tense relationships with her children and their families, who she correctly perceives to be largely uncaring and manipulative.

Let's Dance gives the reader insight into the mind of Serena Burley who is writing up a journal, usually during the early hours of the morning. Serena's children, Robert and Isabel, have decided that 'Serena's erratically developing dementia' (Hegarty 1996: 2) is making it increasingly difficult for them to allow her to continue living alone in her large, isolated country house. Interwoven with the events in the story which include descriptions of Serena's eccentric behaviour and dress are excerpts from her journal allowing readers inside access to her one way of symbolically attempting to preserve the threatened self. In the following passage Serena reflects on the turmoil of her inner life:

> If she had a tape recorder . . . she would be able to say exactly what this condition was like. It was like the nightmare of an operation where the patient is merely drugged, not anaesthetized, rendered immobile and helpless in the face of hideous pain and the knowledge that the surgeon is removing the wrong leg. Or trying to push the baby back in. The image made her cry and giggle at the same time and reminded her that there was no time for crying. Crying only served to eclipse this hour into more of the bumbling confusion that filled the day, apart from those crucial

minutes, sometimes a whole thirty at a time, when she could control the clouds and make them move away from the sun.

(Hegarty 1996: 22)

The essence of symbolic interactionism is the conceptualization of human life as a process. The idea of process implies human experience as a kind of reflexive ebb and flow rather than an undeviating movement in one direction. Serena's confusion, in this respect like Archie's, is not a blanket condition but has emerged 'erratically'. As her journals show, she moves in and out of control of her writing and is aware of the change in her perceptions and her ability to exercise self-control. For her children she is both a problem to be dutifully resolved and the source of mixed feelings of love, embarrassment and anxiety.

Stories

As a product of the creative imagination fiction offers both writers and readers a resource for reflecting upon ageing as symbolic interaction. Mary Stuart (1998: 149) has drawn a parallel between writing and the emergence of the self as a process in everyday life:

> Writing is a process of social interaction. In writing we imagine our reader, we write *to* someone or something. . . . Imagining the reader is a vital component of being able to write. As I write this, I have some notion of who 'you' are. . . . You too will have been imagining me as you read, and I begin to see myself 'anew' as the writing develops.

Writing is therefore an interactive process in certain respects similar to the processes of interaction through which identity is created in everyday life. Just as the writer symbolically expresses the self on a page (either a version of his or her own self or the self of a fictitious character), so in everyday life the self is brought symbolically to life in interaction with other people. In this sense the lived self and the self of fiction are both narratives of stories. The interactionist Ken Plummer has detected an affinity between storytelling and the work of sociology (and, we can add, gerontology), describing human beings as '*homo narrans*' or 'narrators and story tellers' (1997: 5). We humans manipulate symbols to make sense of the world because we live in 'a vast flow of ever-changing' interactions: 'Through symbols and languages, we are able to reflect upon ourselves and others . . . we work and worry, pray and play, love and hate; and *all the time we are telling stories* about our pasts, our presents, and our futures' (Plummer 1997: 20).

For Plummer, stories can be described as 'joint actions' and storytelling can be located 'at the heart of our symbolic interactions'. Other sociologists have highlighted the importance of books as a source of information and guidance about life, especially when it becomes problematic. To borrow from Erving Goffman it can be argued that we live in a 'literally-defined world' (1968: 38) and we may well turn to fiction for information about other people who appear to share the same condition or situation as ourselves. When Barbara Pym's Letty, 'an unashamed reader of novels' retires, she goes to the library

to look for a book 'which reflected her own sort of life' although she is dis-
appointed to find that 'the position of an unmarried, unattached, ageing
woman is of no interest whatever to the writer of modern fiction' (Pym 1994:
6–7). *Quartet in Autumn*, the novel from which I have taken this quotation,
was first published in 1977, and novels about the situation of Letty are now
much more common. For one, we are fortunate in having Barbara Pym's own
work. Almost 20 years later Doris Lessing's Sarah Durham, at the age of 65,
picks up a book of memoirs written by a society woman, a former beauty,
when she had grown older:

> A strange thing, Sarah thought, that she had picked the book up. Once,
> she would never have opened a book by an old person: nothing to do
> with her, she would have felt. But what could be odder than the way
> that books which chime with one's condition or stage in life insinuate
> themselves into one's hand?
>
> (Lessing 1996: 4)

Unlike Letty, Sarah is not looking for fiction, however, the quest for affinity
between the printed symbols in a book and the personal experience of everyday life is the same.

As noted in the outline of symbolic interactionism above, fiction can be a
valuable asset to anyone who wishes to understand the interplay between the
personal and social aspects of the ageing process. Of course it has to be remembered that there are significant variations in the treatment of ageing in fiction.
Authorial styles vary and, as we shall see in the discussion of five variations in
stories of ageing below, novels as a literary form also vary in the depth and style
of treatment they give to later life. For the moment this claim may be illustrated with reference to Penelope Lively's *Spiderweb*, published in 1998.

The title *Spiderweb* clearly suggests a delicate network connecting the person
at the centre of the web, who is called Stella Brentwood, to the past, the present
and the future. Stella has recently retired to a cottage in Somerset but the difference between Stella and other professional unmarried women of her social
class is her former occupation: she has spent her entire working life as an
anthropologist studying village communities in the Nile Delta, Malta, Orkney
and the inner city. She consciously draws, therefore, on her professional language to define her own situation and to make plans for the future:

> She was sixty-five, apparently. This totemic number had landed her here.
> Having spent much time noting and interpreting complex rites of passage
> in alien societies, she now found herself subject to one of the implacable
> rules of her own: stop working, get old.
>
> In other societies the likes of her would be variously seen as valuable
> repositories of knowledge, as objects of pity and respect, or as economic
> encumbrances ripe for disposal. Exempt from such extremes, she could
> define her own position. She could be as she wished, do as she liked.
>
> (Lively 1998: 15)

As a professional observer Stella feels free to 'define her own position' in the
symbolic spiderweb of time and space. She observes around her the signs of
ageing in others such as her friend Richard and carefully, as an anthropologist,

gathers data concerning the new environment in which she has chosen to spend her later life. As she settles into her cottage she rereads her research notebooks and is reminded of her former self and the ways her relationships with other people have changed over the years. Looking back to her field trip to Orkney when she was young, she recalls Alan Scarth, whose offer of marriage she refused. In memory he has not changed:

> When Stella thought now of those months, they had still that sense of a continuous present. And Alan Scarth was frozen in her head as he was then – that fiery, potent giant of a man in the prime of his life. Herself she could not see, because that Stella was eclipsed entirely by subsequent Stellas and above all by the Stella of today, who confronted her from the mirror, features distorted by age, body softened and sagging. Very occasionally, she would be shocked to think that he also, if he was out there still, must now be thus.
>
> (Lively 1998: 193)

In this story of ageing, Stella is aware of herself as having lived a number of selves in her spiderweb of life. The novel is an in-depth description and analysis of one person's efforts to come to terms with retirement and her future life. This is achieved through allowing the reader access to Stella's subjective world where she compares her self with those around her in the process of deciding how to live. In this sense it is a novel of an age-consciousness which derives its meaning from the imaginative realization of changing places, cultures and relationships. In comparison, the character of Gran, the cowed mother of the domineering Karen Hiscox who lives down the road, serves as an almost stereotypical image of an abused, neglected and confused old age. The reader knows that whatever happens in the future, Stella will not end up in this situation. The distance separating these two images of ageing could hardly be greater. 'All novels', suggests Alison Light, 'whether they mean to or not, give us a medley of different voices, languages and positions . . . novels not only speak from their cultural moment but take issue with it, imagining new versions of its problems. . . .' (1991: 2).

Five variations on a theme

The stories I have used in writing this book have been grouped in this section, not as watertight and definitive categories, but as five variations. These are provisional and inevitably artificial because there is often, as is to be expected, some overlap. Inevitably certain titles can be included under more than one heading. The overall principles of selection are, first, the degree of centrality of ageing to the story (the role of ageing in the narrative), and second, the interpretation of the ageing process. My basic aim is simply to highlight the value of fiction as an aid to understanding the interactional variations in the experience of ageing: namely, the interplay between body and self, self and others, objects, places and spaces, and some of the risks to which these are exposed in later life.

Differences in emphasis and interpretation reflected in the five variations come together in a number of ways to form the cultural resources from which the subjective meaning of ageing as a process is configured. In stories of ageing, themes and variations differ in emphasis and structure according to the particular kind of story that is written and the intentions of the author. Novels which follow the lives of the central characters through from early life to old age (for example, Pat Barker's *The Century's Daughter*) or which trace the biographical connections between events in the past and the quality of life in the present (examples include Barbara Ewing's *The Actresses* and Angela Huth's *Land Girls*) obviously offer a more intensely focused interpretation of ageing than those where the older characters are simply incidental figures in a landscape, or where ageing is an incidental point of reference in a sequence of events.

I have therefore grouped the stories I have drawn from to make this book as five variations on the main theme of symbolic interaction between body, self and society. I use the term 'theme' to suggest that these are not definitive nor exclusive categories of fiction but are listed experimentally in order to display some of the key variations in the ways in which the experience of ageing is shaped in the human imagination. Indeed I hope readers will not feel bound by these themes but encouraged to compile their own versions. Variations 1 to 5 below are suggestive rather than prescriptive and are listed simply as a guide to the range of stories I have used to illustrate a processual or interactionist approach to ageing. As previously noted, the range reflects variations in the space taken up by ageing as a theme in each novel (ranging from central in Variation 1 to peripheral in Variation 5) and the intensity of interest in subjective experience and social interaction between characters in various age groups. Clearly a novel where the age identity of the main character is the central theme, such as Doris Lessing's *Love Again*, will offer a much more sustained description and interpretation of the experience of ageing than one where the older characters are more incidental to the narrative. An example of the latter is Reginald Hill's murder mystery *On Beulah Height*. Yet even when older characters are comparatively incidental figures or used basically as a device to add momentum to the plot or social background to the narrative they may have something significant to reveal about the meanings which are culturally ascribed to ageing and the implications of these symbolic constructions for the subjective experience of growing older. Very often such figures are simply routine stereotypical representations of ageing but they have been included because stereotypes have been shown to play a significant part in the shaping of collective and subjective age consciousness (Featherstone and Hepworth 1993; Bytheway 1995). In other words, stereotypes work precisely *because* they reflect and confirm taken-for-granted ideas about ageing and older people.

The variations are as follows:

Variation 1

The interest of the writer is in *one central character, often the narrator, who is ageing*. Age identity or a subjective age consciousness is central in such novels which often involve an extensive life review.

Examples include Thea Astley's *Coda*, Anita Brookner's *A Private View*, Eva Figes' *Ghosts*, Anthony Gilbert's *The Spinster's Secret*, Doris Lessing's *Love Again*, Penelope Lively's *Spiderweb*, James Long's *Ferney*, Julian Rathbone's *Blame*

Hitler, Vita Sackville-West's *All Passion Spent*, Jane Smiley's *At Paradise Gate*, and Henry Sutton's *Gorleston*.

Variation 2

The writer's attention is focused on a *small group of older characters*. Such a collection of older people may, for example be living in retirement at the seaside as in Henry Sutton's *Gorleston* or Stanley Middleton's *Necessary Ends*; or they may be gathered together in a particular building such as a private hotel, or some form of residential accommodation. In stories of life in a residential group (for instance Elizabeth Taylor's *Mrs Palfrey At The Claremont* or Paul Bailey's *At The Jerusalem*) the age identity of one particular character may be central but there is the additional interest of networks of interpersonal relationships, tensions and conflicts within the group and also with people living in the outside world.

Examples range from Kingsley Amis' *Ending Up*, Roy Clarke's *Gala Week*, Marika Cobbold's *Guppies for Tea*, Kathleen Conlon's *Face Values*, Christopher Hope's *Serenity House* and Alan Isler's *The Prince of West End Avenue*.

Variation 3

The emphasis here is on *family interaction*. In particular the intense and highly emotive forms of interpersonal interaction that take place between different generations of members of a particular family and the influence of these relationships on the ageing process.

Examples include Thea Astley's *Coda*, Nina Bawden's *Family Money*, Pat Barker's *The Century's Daughter*, Robert Barnard's *Posthumous Papers*, Nicci French's *The Memory Game*, Margaret Forster's *Have The Men Had Enough?* and *The Seduction of Mrs Pendlebury*, Frances Hegarty's *Let's Dance*, Penelope Lively's *The Road to Lichfield* and *Passing On*, Francois Mauriac's *The Knot of Vipers*, Deborah Moggach's *Close Relations*, David Renwick's *One Foot in The Grave* and Joanna Trollope's *The Men and the Girls*.

Variation 4

The stories in this variation are, like those in Variation 3, concerned with age-related interpersonal interaction. The main difference is that these stories are less concerned with close relationships between family members and are more interested in *age-related relationships outside the family situation* between friends, and, on a more formal social level, with strangers.

Examples include Celia Dale's *A Helping Hand* and *Sheep's Clothing*, Barbara Ewing's *The Actresses*, Angela Huth's *Land Girls*, Stanley Middleton's *Beginning to End* and Julian Rathbone's *Intimacy*.

Variation 5

Here, the interest of the story is not so directly focused on the qualities of interpersonal interaction among younger/older people but on *descriptions of older characters and of the ageing process*.

Examples include Philip Caveney's *Skin Flicks*, Agatha Christie's *Hercule Poirot's Christmas* and *Curtain: Poirot's Last Case*, Marika Cobbold's *A Rival Creation*, Colin Dexter's *The Wench is Dead*, John Harvey's *Easy Meat*, James Herriot's *If Only They Could Talk*, Reginald Hill's *Exit Lines* and *Recalled to Life*, Laurie Lee's *Cider With Rosie*, Ruth Rendell's *Simisola* and Kathleen Rowntree's *Mr Brightly's Evening Off*.

Discussion

In Variations 1 to 4 the ageing of a main character, a family group, a small group of characters or a group brought together in a distinctive place is the central theme of the narrative. These are stories which are directly focused on specific qualities of the experience of ageing as such. In Variation 5 ageing is not usually the main theme of the story, but older characters make an interesting contribution to the flow of the narrative or a noteworthy reference to ageing appears. This treatment can range from the incidental, where older people are introduced, usually stereotypically as background figures, to the author's use of an older character as a peg on which to hang a narrative.

Ageing can be also introduced to maintain continuity between one novel and another in a series, or within a particular novel to add to the credibility of the characters and to give the impression of the chronological flow of 'real life'. A good example of this practice can be found in some of the crime fiction of Reginald Hill. In *Recalled to Life* a background theme to this murder mystery is the difficulty Inspector Peter Pascoe's wife Ellie is having with her ageing parents. Earlier in this chapter I quoted a conversation from one of Hill's previous novels in his Dalziel and Pascoe series, *Exit Lines*, where Pascoe's mother-in-law tells him about her anxiety over her husband's erratic behaviour. But time has passed (*Recalled to Life*) and Ellie's father Archie has been diagnosed as suffering from Alzheimer's and 'is in a Home now' (Hill 1993: 211) Ellie's worries over her father's state of mind have been replaced by anxiety about her mother who is herself afraid she is becoming confused like her husband. Over the phone Ellie explains to Peter:

> after what she went through with Dad, she doesn't want to know, so she hides it from herself by hiding it from me. I noticed she was going to bed later, and later and when I nagged her into talking about it, it came out that often when she wakes up in the morning, she doesn't know where she is or even who she is, and that's making her scared to go to sleep.
>
> (Hill 1993: 271–2)

After a consultation with a specialist it is discovered that although she is suffering from high blood pressure and arthritis, 'Ninety per cent of her forgetfulness is probably caused by medication, and the other ten per cent by worry' (Hill 1993: 376–7).

The ageing of Ellie's parents is not a contributory factor to any of the murders Dalziel and Pascoe have to solve, but it provides a line of continuity in the domestic life of Pascoe, adding a recognizably mundane dimension to his character and sustaining the illusion that he is a 'real' human being with many of the worries that afflict at least some of the readers.

Examples of the background stereotyping of older people in fiction are numberless. As I mentioned above, this device is often used in stories in Variation 1 where an in-depth treatment of an ageing individual is the main concern. Stereotypes may be used in such novels as contrasting figures to point up the individuality or unusual qualities of the main character, as is the case in Barbara Vine's *The Brimstone Wedding* where Jenny, a young carer in a private home for the wealthy, perceives Stella to be quite different from the other residents who are seen in contrast to be decrepit and inarticulate. A close relationship develops between Stella and Jenny during the course of which Stella emerges as a highly complex character with a convoluted personal story. The interaction between the two characters develops the identities of both.

In Christopher Hope's *Serenity House*, the central character Max, who we shall meet again later, is regarded by the owner of the home as a cut above the rest. A man who despite his years, and the evidence of decline in his appearance, still displays vestiges of the 'gentleman'.

Lastly, in an incident from Marika Cobbold's *Guppies For Tea*, Amelia Lindsey has taken her grandmother, Selma, on a taxi ride. Selma is becoming more and more confused but readers are aware by page 111 that her confusion is a fluctuating condition and she has a close relationship with Amelia whom she helped to raise. Selma is therefore a rounded character whose ageing is in this novel highly individualized:

> When the car stopped at a red light, an old woman, her thick legs disappearing inside dumpy suede boots, a plastic rain cover tied round her whispy grey hair, hastened across.
>
> 'Goodness me, some people are hideous,' Selma remarked cheerfully. She sat there, whiskery-chinned, and missing her teeth, her cardigan spotted with stains, and yet she looked at the woman at the crossing with gleeful disapproval. Selma had been beautiful. Thank God, Amelia thought, that in her mind she still is.
>
> (Cobbold 1993: 111)

As readers of this story, we are invited to see Selma through Amelia's eyes and to sympathize with Amelia's determined efforts to ensure her grandmother comes to a dignified end, even though the staff of the expensive private home to which she is admitted at the beginning of the story soon find her very difficult to handle and request her removal. The figure of the old woman on the crossing also allows us an insight into Selma's inability to identify with the social category 'old age' and the persistence in her own mind of the image of a former self. Fortunately for Selma, Amelia shares her awareness of this former self and can continue to confirm it in symbolic interaction.

We noted earlier how Barbara Pym's Letty (*Quartet in Autumn*) deplored the limited number of stories about women in her age group and situation, and we also noted an increase in such stories since that novel first appeared in 1977. Stories in Variation 1, where interest is concentrated on one central character who is ageing, appear to be on the increase (Gullette 1988, 1993). Older characters, it is argued in literary gerontology, are being moved by their authors from a marginal position in fiction to centre stage. When 'they appear in fiction old people are now much less likely to be afforded only the passing glance or minor role that was customary in the past . . .' (Rooke 1992: 241). I have listed above a number of novels in this variation where the author focuses directly on the engagement of a character with ageing. In stories of this kind the author is usually preoccupied with the inner life and personal perspective of the central character (for example, Lessing's *Love Again*); and the experiences imagined may be conveyed in terms of positive 'progress' narratives of later life or negative 'decline narratives', or a combination of both (Gullette 1988: xvi). But in all cases the reader is invited to engage sympathetically with the subjective perspective of the main character who is directly engaging with the biographical implications of growing older.

In this respect the main character in stories in Variation 1 becomes the expert on ageing. In a lively incident in Bernice Rubens' novel *The Waiting Game* about 'The Hollyhocks', a 'Home for the Aged' (Rubens 1997: 3), the matron invites 'an expert on ageing to come to talk to her residents' (p. 200). As she correctly anticipates, the prospect of a talk on ageing turns out to be very popular. But when he arrives the expert, Mr Roberts, is 25 years old and greeted with an atmosphere of hostility and contempt. Sensing this he defuses the tension by acknowledging from the start that 'everybody in this room knows a damn sight more about ageing than I do' (p. 201). He then proceeds to inform his audience that he has interviewed hundreds of 'people like your good selves' (p. 201) and asks them to help him by sharing their opinions and wisdom. This gambit does the trick, though unfortunately only for a brief interlude following which arguments break out between the residents and personal disputes and rivalries are revealed. The talk ends in chaos: 'nobody wanted to listen to Mr Roberts any more and his twenty-odd-year-old geriatric experience. Mr Roberts was more than happy to oblige them, having decided that in future he would address his geriatric lecture to classes of sixth-formers' (p. 205).

An even more sardonic version of the 'knowing insider' can be found in Christopher Meade's comic character Betty Spital, 'Pensioner, Activist and Radical Granny', who dispenses an assortment of home truths about the ageing experience in *The Thoughts of Betty Spital*. Meade's send-up of handbooks on positive ageing includes a chapter on 'The New Gerontology' where we can read a dismissive reflection on the word 'gerontology', which is derived from:

> the Greek 'geron', meaning old, mature, wise, beyond reproach and 'ology' meaning you can write books about it, run evening classes in it, appear on TV and radio talking about it – and possibly end up as a professor of it, till death or early retirement, in some nice cosy university somewhere.
>
> (Meade 1989: 36)

Stories of ageing I have included in Variation 1 often narrate a history of the self as they explore in a form of 'life review' the route the central character has taken to arrive at her or his present situation and assume a particular identity. This is a central issue in Barbara Vine's *The Brimstone Wedding*. Stella is dying of cancer but guards a closely kept secret concerning her previous life. As mentioned above, a close rapport develops between her and

Jenny, her carer to whom she gradually discloses information about her personal history she is unwilling to share with her family. The idea that older people's past lives are not necessarily an open book to their close relations provides the mystery to hold the reader's attention and simultaneously offers a sensitive picture of a care relationship and the subjective experience of Stella in coping with residential care.

A similar process of disclosing the history of an older person's inner self unfolds in quite a different novel, May Sarton's *Mrs Stevens Hears the Mermaids Singing*. Hilary Stevens, a famous poet, comes to terms with herself during the course of an interview with a younger man and woman for a literary magazine. After the interview is over Hilary goes for a walk with Mar, a young man with whom she has become friendly:

> His eyes looked very blue, and for a second Hilary envied him, envied that masculine power, that youth, the *animal* in him.
>
> 'I'm an old woman,' she said heavily, and this time with disgust. 'But when I was your age, or a little younger maybe, I wanted to be a boy. Part of me just stayed back there, and you can laugh if you must – it might be appropriate! – but it was (and *is*) that boy in me who wrote the poems. So I have kept him close to me, for better or worse, and perhaps justified my way of life in the light of his immature eyes.'
>
> (Sarton 1993: 217)

In Variation 2 the centre of attention is the processes of interaction between a small number of older characters often gathered together in a particular place. The tragi-comedy of power struggles in later life is a prominent theme in fiction of this kind. The ageing body can be deployed in terms of differences of location, gender, social class and risk to create tension and human interest. Stories about a group of older people provide an opportunity to describe variations in character and the complex relationships, tensions and conflicts between a number of people living under the same roof. This was the explicit intention of Kingsley Amis when he wrote *Ending Up*.

Another dramatic value for stories of ageing is that these clusters of characters have often not come together through an entirely free personal choice. The writer can create interest by portraying individual variations between characters who may unwillingly share the common experience of old age. The author can show that the physical frailties which accompany ageing do not eliminate social hierarchies, competition for status, sexual desire or disruptive emotions such as anger, jealousy, envy and resentment. In other words, people are not transformed into a different kind of human being simply because they are chronologically and physically old and end up in residential accommodation. Nor are they necessarily transformed into nicer, kinder or more benign beings typified by the greetings-card stereotype of the cheery 'granny' or grandfather.

In Variation 3 the interest in interaction between older and younger characters often revolves around a family setting. Examples include two novels by Margaret Forster: *The Seduction of Mrs Pendlebury*, where a relationship develops between younger neighbours and an older couple, and *Have the Men Had Enough?* where the central character, 'grandma', is seen through the eyes of the other family members for whom she is becoming increasingly a problem as she grows more physically dependent and confused.

In the case of Mrs Pendlebury, readers are admitted to Rose's confused subjective world and can empathize with her unstable vision of life on the outside in sharp contrast to the perceptions of her husband Stanley and her younger neighbour, Alice. This comparative perspective allows Rose to be rescued from anonymity or collective stereotyping. Her younger neighbours think that both Rose and her husband are 'pathetic' (Forster 1978: 199) and are determined they will not end up the same. But for readers who have become much more intimately acquainted with Stanley and Rose as individuals with personal histories, ageing is a much more complex process involving a fluctuation between positive and negative experiences and emotions.

Some of the stories in Variation 4 vary somewhat from those included in Variations 1–3 in so far as the main interest may not be directly concerned with the processes of interaction that socially construct age identities in everyday life. In this variation older characters may be used as a device for getting a story going and this can include the ploy of them as victims of murder. An example of an older victim in a murder mystery is Ann Granger's *A Word After Dying*. In another murder mystery, Marianne Macdonald's *Ghost Walk*, events are triggered off by the appearance of a scruffy old man, Tom Ashe, who seems to be a vagrant. But, as the story unfolds, information about his life accumulates and, in sharp contrast to other older figures in the background of the story, he assumes a complex identity. When, for example, he is visited in hospital by the narrator (Dido Hoare, a young bookselling private investigator) after being found unconscious in a shop doorway, Dido finds it difficult at first to separate him out from the other old men on the ward:

> In here, they were mostly old men who lay propped motionless in the white beds, staring at a shrunken world. A television set high on the wall was broadcasting a morning chat show, but the sound had been turned to an inaudible rumble, so that the faces on the screen mouthed and smiled meaninglessly. I felt a moment of panic, wondering whether I was going to recognise Ashe in this gathering of old bones.
>
> (Macdonald 1997: 12)

The interrelationship of place and the identity of older people will be discussed in greater detail in Chapter 4, but for the moment the 'shrunken world' of the hospital mirrors the collective shrunken status of the patients who, in contrast with the individualized Ashe, are institutionalized into insignificance. Their anonymity is used to highlight Ashe who is selectively perceived as a recognizable individual and not merely another old man.

When reading any of the five variations of stories of ageing I have provisionally drawn upon, the relationship of author to text and reader to author and text is always complex and by no means certain. But what I want to stress is the role of the author's imagination in giving access to a range of perspectives on the experience of ageing which are not always possible in conventional gerontological research. In fiction the possibility exists of exploring facets of the ageing process which are often inaccessible to the external observer of everyday life, however skilled he or she may be.

In stories of ageing the experience of growing older may be imagined from a number of perspectives. Because writers are free to invent characters with identifiable bodies and selves, relationships, situations, risks and futures they can display aspects of the ageing process that may be deliberately concealed from public view or accessible to researchers only after considerable effort and expense. As I have tried to show, stories vary in the depth of their treatment of ageing but in their varying forms they are a valuable additional source of data for those who wish to understand the multi-faceted experience of growing older.

However, this is not to say that in the world of fiction anything goes. Fiction is never the unfettered reign of the imagination because, like any symbolic medium, it has to work within certain rules if the author is to communicate effectively with the audience. There is then a creative tension between the conventions of fiction – what the readership will expect and tolerate – and the imagination of the author. Readers bring their beliefs and values to the process of reading and are free within the limits of their imaginations to make their own interpretations of the meanings of stories. As Cole has noted in relation to meaning, 'no matter how carefully one defines or analyses it, there can never be an objective, predefined formula capable of externally grasping the meaning of *meaning*. As self-defining and self-interpreting animals, we humans must enter into our own webs of meaning to understand ourselves' (1992: xviii).

Because stories are products of the creative imagination they are inevitably about the ways writers and their readers imagine later life and in this respect they have a point of contact with reality. A good example from popular crime fiction is Agatha Christie's Miss Marple who is, of course, an idealized image of the genteel spinster living quietly in a stereotypical English village. I remember some years ago including a reference to Miss Marple in a talk about the sociology of ageing and a number of people came up to me at the end and said how pleased they were that I had introduced this well-known figure into a talk which consisted mainly of less familiar academic analysis. It was not, of course, that they believed that Miss Marple ever existed in reality, but that certain elements of her imagined role, her appearance, personal style, biography and social situation, have a strong appeal to the imagination and are thereby interwoven with the mundane reality of everyday life. And Agatha Christie herself suggested that some of Miss Marple's characteristics were derived from her direct observations of some of the older members of her family. Miss Marple was:

> the sort of old lady who would have been rather like some of my grandmother's Ealing cronies – old ladies whom I have met in so many villages where I have gone to stay as a girl. Miss Marple was not in any way a picture of my grandmother; she was far more fussy and spinsterish than my grandmother ever was. But the thing she did have in common with her – though a cheerful person, she always expected the worst of everyone and everything, and was, with almost frightening accuracy, usually proved right.

> (Christie 1978: 449–50)

The widespread appeal of the Miss Marple stories, as bestselling novels, in film and TV dramatizations, suggests that they occupy a positive place in the collective imagination. On the level of the imaginary, Miss Marple reveals the possibility of a superior role for the wisdom of the older woman in modern society. Stories of ageing do not therefore have to be factually accurate in order to shape and give meaning to everyday experience. We swim, says A.A. Berger, 'in a sea of stories and tales that we hear or read or listen to or see. . . .' (1997: 1). Stories of ageing involve an interplay between the external reality of everyday experience and our internal subjective worlds of desires, anxieties, fears, and fantasies. In our private imaginary worlds we reflect on the ideas about ageing circulating around us in the wider culture. And these reflections are intimately related to our powers of self-expression and deepest emotions; it is important to remember that novels help people to *feel* as well as think.

Because it is now accepted that there is no single 'right' way of interpreting fiction and that novels are open to a variety of interpretations, there is greater freedom for all of us, as writers and readers, to look for ways of giving symbolic form to the experience of ageing and to try to explore the connections between our own subjective experiences and those of others. To make use, in other words, of the connections between self and others which are central to symbolic interactionist analysis. Paula Crimmens, who specializes in training people who work with older people, finds Michael Ignatieff's novel *Scar Tissue* about dementia as the loss of self both 'wonderful' and misleading because she does not consider that a personality changed by illness means a loss of self: 'I have never met anyone without a self. I would not know what that looked like. And if we say this person has no sense of self with whom are we interacting and where has their sense of self gone? How is this going to affect the way we treat them?' (Crimmens 1998: 142).

Whatever variation they may adopt, stories of ageing always invite us to relate self to others; to imagine our own ageing and the implications of this mental vision for 'the way we treat' other older people. There is a sense in which stories of ageing never really stand on neutral ground and at this point I shall conclude the provisional discussion of their five variations. For the rest of the book I shall draw selectively from the literature to follow through some of the connections we imaginatively make between body, self, and society in order to make sense of the ageing of ourselves and of others.

2

Body and self

Self as process

From the symbolic interactionist perspective the self is not seen as some kind of personal property we are born with, created in advance of our awareness of it and housed 'inside' the body, but a living process which changes throughout the life course. The ageing process is itself evidence that change is a fundamental feature of the human condition: individuals do not remain unaltered as they grow older. But three qualifying statements should also be made at this point. First, the emphasis on process as continuous change does not imply that changes to the self are necessarily dramatic or consciously experienced. Many of the changes associated with ageing are on a very small scale and cumulative in effect.

Second, the idea of the self as an emergent dynamic process does not mean that there is no such thing as a 'core self' or sense of continuous personal identity. The division of the self into the two dimensions, private and public, acknowledges the existence of individual self-consciousness or a personal sense of a stable and continuous identity (Cohen 1994). Just to give one fictional example, Stella in Barbara Vine's *The Brimstone Wedding* retires to her room in the residential home to dictate her secret past to a tape recorder. To ensure privacy she puts a chair under the door handle and she also finds security in the popular belief that older people often talk to themselves:

> It's possible that one of the people here, pausing outside my door, in innocence or deliberately to listen, can hear my voice if not what I'm saying. Fortunately, in one way I'm no longer able to speak very loudly [Stella is terminally ill with lung cancer]. I don't really mind if they do hear a continuous murmur from inside. They will only think I'm talking to myself and that won't surprise them. Everyone here except Genevieve [Jenny, the young care assistant with whom she has become friendly]

takes it for granted the residents have softening of the brain or are dropping into a second childhood.

(Vine 1996: 55)

As Cohen has pointed out, and as we shall explore further, one of the main
tasks for people in later life is to hold onto the self and to resist the 'attacks
made on its integrity' (Cohen 1994: 99).

Third, to return to the previous discussion of the freedom of readers to
interpret stories in the light of their own experience, the possibility of realiz-
ing change in later life is inevitably determined by the cultural and social
resources available. Just as novelists have to write within a framework of
narrative conventions if their stories are to make sense to readers, so older
people have to express themselves and make their own sense of ageing in
relation to the situations in which they live. In this respect fictional representations of ageing, as we have already noted, often reveal a wide gulf
between public images and definitions of later life and the subjective experience of the individual.

Dorothy Jerrome (1992), who has observed the differences between the
public and private 'faces' of older women in her study of clubs for older people
on the south coast of England, has recorded some of the ways in which older
people negotiate between themselves the meanings of the experience of
ageing. In the interactive processes revealed in this particular study, each individual draws on the cultural resources of a 'church club' – beliefs that life is
a spiritual journey to a better world and that religion offers compensations
for the aches, pains and illnesses associated with old age – to make personal
sense of growing older. They are not entirely free to make up their own ideas
about ageing but they do have some freedom of choice: members of these
clubs 'enjoy a degree of latitude in the construction of ageing identities'
(Jerrome 1992: 190).

Stories of ageing work in their various ways within the 'latitude' to which
Jerrome refers and what Gullette has described as 'the fundamental condition
of possibility' (1988: xvi). As symbolic representations of life they show how
ageing becomes more than a biological process and is transformed in relationship with other people into a meaningful experience. Throughout the rest of
this book we shall see how fictional representations of ageing, drawn from
the five variations outlined in Chapter 1, display this symbolic interplay in
action. With these pointers in mind I now turn to a discussion of the symbolic interactionist approach to the question of the body and the self.

Body and self

One of the most interesting and challenging facts about human ageing is that
it raises important questions about the nature of the relationship between the
body, the self and society. And these questions are not merely academic, they
are of profound personal concern to us all.

There is no doubt (at least in western civilizations) that one of the most disturbing images of later life is that of physical decline. Indeed, the negative
emotions associated with ageing are prompted by the idea of the deeply

ageing body (Elias 1985). The problem of the painful and ageing body is poignantly described by Pat Barker in *Union Street*, a series of stories about seven women who live on Union Street in a working-class area of a depressed town in the North of England. The last chapter is about Alice Bell, a woman aged over 70, living alone in seriously run-down accommodation and struggling with her ailing body after a stroke:

> She turned the right side of her body away from people so that all her movements became crab-like. She could not wash and dress herself. She could not get around very well.
>
> Words still clotted on her tongue whenever she became confused, though after the first few weeks her speech was generally easier to understand. Only she still had difficulty with the endings of words. They tended to get left off or to turn up attached to other words. Still more disconcertingly, she found herself thinking one thing and saying another, not realising, until she heard herself that she was talking nonsense. People, seeing that she found speech difficult, behaved as if she was deaf. Since, in fact, her hearing had become abnormally acute, their braying voices exploded inside her head, sending splinters of pain to every part.
>
> But she did not give in. No, would not, not if she was brought down to the gutter.
>
> (Barker 1982: 249)

Here is a description of some of the ways in which the ageing of the body intrudes in the process of communicating the self to others. But it is also much more. First, this process is individualized in the character of Alice Bell who is by no means, even when her bodily condition is so graphically described, some anonymous symbol of biological human fate. The key lines in this quotation are the last two: Alice 'did not give in'. Nor does she. Despite her pitifully reduced condition, Alice refuses to wait to be taken away from her home, struggles into her clothes and staggers out into the freezing cold to the park where she is forced to sit down on a bench. And there she dies:

> But there was a child there, now, a girl, who, standing with the sun behind her, seemed almost to be a gift of the light. At first she was afraid, the child had come so suddenly. Then – not afraid. They sat beside each other; they talked. The girl held out her hand. The withered hand and the strong young hand met and joined. There was silence. Then it was time for them both to go.
>
> (Barker 1982: 265)

Pat Barker's Alice is a picture of dignified suffering. Of the maintenance of the self against the odds of a relentlessly declining body and the efforts of her son Tom and his wife Doreen to put her into a 'Home'. From their point of view she is becoming totally dependent and is hallucinating. The reader, however, is invited to identify with Alice's definition of the situation and her determination to leave the world on her own terms.

Pat Barker has created another example of the struggle of the body with the self in *Another World*. Geordie, a working-class man, aged 101, widowed and now not far from death, makes one last supreme effort to spruce himself up for a visit from Helen. She is a younger woman, an academic who previously interviewed him about his memories of being a soldier in the First World War. During these interviews a sympathetic relationship developed and Helen is now visiting Geordie for what we know will be the last time. Nick, his grandson, becomes aware that Geordie has struggled out of bed and spruced himself up because he is in love with Helen. The reader sees the interaction between Geordie and Helen through Nick's eyes:

> Geordie's sitting up, incredibly erect, though a few minutes ago he'd been slumped over his swollen belly. The suspicious areas of brightness in his cheeks are more clearly marked than ever.

Helen and Geordie exchange kisses and talk:

> They're sitting together easily and yet intently, still holding hands, and suddenly Nick realizes something that's probably been staring him in the face for years. Geordie's in love with Helen, in love with a woman sixty years younger than himself, hopelessly, helplessly and no doubt at times humiliatingly in love, and has been ever since he met her. This is why he's achieved this minor resurrection from the dead. This is why it matters so much that he should be shaved and dressed, and that the house should not smell of his decaying body.
>
> (Barker 1998: 240)

Barker does not spare us detailed descriptions of the physical decay of Geordie's cancer of the bowel but she also allows us to see him, through the eyes of Helen and Nick who love him in their different ways, as a man of dignity. Like Alice Bell, Geordie is not simply a decaying body, just another sick old man, but a richly complex self with a long history in which traumatic memories of the First World War play a significant role.

While there can be no doubt that the body 'is the bedrock of the *real*', and when we think about old age 'we must think about the increasing vulnerability of the body' (Woodward 1991: 23), it is also clear that the self continues its symbolic struggle to survive old age. The separation of the inner subjective Alice from her dilapidated and malfunctioning body at the end of her story, and Geordie's temporary subordination of his intrusive body at the end of his are celebrations of the symbolic nature of selfhood. They are examples of the liberatory power of symbols mentioned in Chapter 1.

For the symbolic interactionist, society always comes first. And yet, paradoxically perhaps, for the symbolic interactionist the body also always comes first. This is because human beings are regarded primarily as biological creatures, subject to biological processes of growth and change. But biology is conceptualized in dynamic interaction with society and culture. Babies are born into a network of social relationships in a state of complete infantile dependence on other humans who have been born before. As tiny infants we are bodies of biologically determined potential which must be stimulated by social interaction to begin to exhibit signs of individual selfhood and to take on a recognizable social identity (children, says Allison James, 'are yet-to-be' – 1995: 61). From our earliest moments in the world the two dimensions of selfhood begin to emerge in interaction with others: personal consciousness of self as separate from other individuals and a social identity created for us by those on whom we are dependent.

According to G.H. Mead (1863–1931), the founding father of symbolic interactionism, the individual sense of selfhood is a feature of the human mind (see, for example, Chappell and Orbach 1986; Burkitt 1991). It is therefore *reflexive* (derived from the stimulus of other people) and *reflective* (it gradually comes into being as conscious independent thought). In this process it is the infant's consciousness of dependence on others which makes consciousness of independent selfhood possible: the one cannot exist without the other. This explains, Mead argued, why throughout life we experience the self as a kind of internal conversation as when, for example, we use the well-known expression 'and so I said to myself.' Much of our inner subjective life is expressed in the form of an internal conversation between ourself and imagined others in our heads. In our heads we often 'hear' the voices of other people, especially family members and close relations. I can without any effort 'hear' the voices of my father and mother which have persisted apparently agelessly long after their deaths. Similarly, Helen, one of the main middle-aged characters in Penelope Lively's *Passing On*, continues to hear the voice of her mother, Dorothy, and to be influenced (in her case, dominated) by her symbolic presence.

These internal conversations have their origins in relationships and conversations in the external world and our ability to reflect gradually emerges as part of the personal self we recognize as our core identity. For Mead the development of language as a symbolic form is the basis of the emergence of the personal and social self. Through the use of language the subjective self can be externalized symbolically in speech and in writing. The separation of the self into two parts makes it possible for us to reflect on the acts of speaking and writing even as we speak and write. Just as we are able to distance ourselves from others so we can distance ourselves from ourselves and monitor our own social performances. Sometimes we are surprised by what we discover. Stella, who was dictating her secret past life into a tape recorder, is disconcerted by the sound of her own voice on playback and thinks 'how much lighter it sounded than she had expected. It sounded light and precise and old-fashioned and *old*' (Vine 1996: 54). Our concern with how we appear to others and to ourselves does not evaporate in later life although it may be impaired by mental or physical illness. Stella, described in *The Brimstone Wedding* as a lively and well-presented woman in spite of the fact she is terminally ill, sees her reaction to the tape recording as vanity: 'She was still vain she thought, even now. Dying, actually dying, she would probably still care how she looked and sounded.' (pp. 54–5).

The names Mead gave to these two interdependent facts of the self were the 'I' and the 'me'. Burkitt explains that the 'me' is the 'unique identity a self develops through seeing its forms in the attitude others take towards it, while the "I" is the subjective attitude of reflection itself, which gazes on both the subjective image of the self and its own responses' (1991: 38). Mead's 'I' is made possible by the human capacity to think independently about external events and to experience the self reflexively as conversation. The human capacity for self-reflection is one important aspect of symbolic liberation from biology we discussed earlier. In Burkitt's words, the 'I' is 'the process of thinking' but there is an important issue of time in this interactive process because 'once the thought is born and becomes tangible, it belongs to the "me". In the inner conversation, the "I" articulates thoughts and the "me" hears them expressed, recognising the voice as its own' (1991: 39).

Because the 'I' exists in the immediate present and can be recalled only as a memory, the 'me' is our memory of what the 'I' said in millions of fleeting moments. Inevitably the 'me' is a memory selectively recalled when we tell stories about events in our lives and about ourselves. Linda Grant (1998) has written movingly about the onset of her mother's dementia and the breakdown of her memory (indicated precisely in the title of her non-fiction book, *Remind Me Who I Am, Again*). The self, she says, 'is not a little person inside the brain, it's a work in progress' (p. 294), and she argues that our lives are essentially stories because they are edited versions of our memories of all the things that have happened to us, transformed into 'a meaningful narrative' (p. 293). If for any reason our own memory lets us down then we become even more reliant on others to help us fill the gaps – and in severe cases of dementia to keep on reminding us who we were and are (Kitwood 1998).

The Meadian analysis of the self as a symbolic construct has clear implications for our understanding of the experience of ageing. In Mead's view the self is not housed in the body but exists in *relation* to it. Because symbolic interactionists envisage the self in the form of a social process, with the potential for change throughout the entire life course, the ageing of the body does not destroy the self though it certainly produces changes in the relationship between body and self. According to this view, the self of a dementing person has not disappeared, but is undergoing a transformation which has multiple causes, including the neuropathological (Lyman 1998; Sabat 1998). To keep the self of the person with dementia socially alive, efforts have to be made by outsiders to help the individual maintain some continuity of identity by reaffirming the past (or 'old') self that she or he may be forgetting in relation to the immediate self ('new') expressed in the present. In extreme cases the person with dementia has apparently lost the internal ability to exercise complete control over his or her story of the self, and the task has to be taken up by outsiders who in effect become the custodians of that person's selfhood (Kitwood 1998).

A central feature of the interactional model of dementia care is the recognition of the role of social approval in the maintenance of self-esteem in later life. The attitudes of others make a significant contribution to the quality of life. In Mead's analysis of the emerging individual identity the infant's growing consciousness of self – the 'I' in relation to the 'me' – is gradually assembled out of an awareness of the ways other people regard her or him. In other words, the attitudes of other people are a kind of living mirror in which the infant initially looks for signs of approval. We learn very quickly how to see ourselves through the eyes of others. The self comes to exist in relationship to the other. The ability to adopt the attitudes of others towards the self does not, however, imply that we as individuals are merely rubber stamps or facsimiles of others. This is the point at which the symbolic elements in reflective and reflexive self-consciousness play a significant part in our awareness of being separate individuals:

Symbols enable individuals to experience and express their attachment to a society or group without compromising their individuality. . . . We may all listen to the same Mahler symphony but hear it differently. We may all participate in the same ritual, pray the same liturgy, speak the same language, but we cannot assume that these social forms convey to us the same meanings.

(Cohen 1994: 19)

The search for meaning in life is therefore a constant process of comparison of self with others. In Andrea Newman's *A Sense of Guilt* (1989), Helen meets her ex-husband Carey whom she has not seen for some time. There is a moment in this encounter when Helen registers Carey's changed appearance. He looks 'much older and heavier' than she remembers, 'and there was far more grey in his hair'. But Helen is not simply a detached observer of Carey's ageing, there is a reflexive moment after Carey has put his hand over hers at the table and 'looked at their hands, and then at her face. He looked old and grey and tired, a man who had come to terms with his situation. She saw her own lost youth in his face and remembered how they had both intended to be famous and rich and in love for ever' (p. 159).

Another reason why in Mead's view human beings are more than the sum total of their relationships is the fact that social life, like biological life, is not static but a processual flux. Burkitt (1991) reminds us that the 'I' is a fleeting expression of the moment and the 'me' a memory in the context of change. Helen's meeting with Carey brings home to her that changes have taken place of which she was not fully aware and she is forced into making a comparison between her memory of the past and their present situation. Another version of reflexive age consciousness can be found in this next example from a story of later life, May Sarton's *As We Are Now*. Caro Spencer has been admitted to Twin Elms nursing home and is brooding over the anger she feels at the treatment she is receiving:

I sometimes think that I feel things more *intensely* than I used to, not less. But I am so afraid of appearing ridiculous. People expect serenity of the old. That is the stereotype, the mask we are expected to put on. But how many old people *are* serene? I have known one or two. My Granny was, but my grandfather, my father's father, became very violent and irascible. I was terrified of him and my father dreaded going to see him. He was forever going to court about some supposed slight or slander.

(Sarton 1992: 81)

Caro's reflection on her experience of 'all the horrors of decay' (Sarton 1992: 80) is a subjective comparison of the changes she observes in her physical appearance and bodily and mental abilities with public stereotypes of ageing and her own particular memories of her grandparents. What is important in this example is the subtle awareness of three temporal perspectives: Caro's memory of her attitude to older people (her grandparents) when she was young, her present awareness (the 'me' of the past) and resentment over her immediate condition (the 'I'). In this comparative symbolization of past, present and prospective future Caro also rejects the idea that she may have anything in common with the other residents of Twin Elms. Like Vine's Stella in Middleton Hall (*The Brimstone Wedding*), and Hope's Max in Serenity House (*Serenity House*), she is a cut above the rest but, more significantly, she cannot bring herself to believe that she shares their condition – old age:

> How expression relieves the mind! I feel quite lively and myself again just because I have managed to write two pages of dissent about old age!
>   Among all the other deprivations here we are deprived of *expression*. The old men slowly atrophy because no one asks them what they feel or why. Could they speak if someone did? And why haven't I tried? I look at them from very far away as if they were in the distance, across a wide river. We have nothing in common. Why pretend that we do?
>
> (Sarton 1992: 81–2)

Moreover, the symbolic act of self-expression in writing reaffirms the independence of Caro's self from others in a similar situation.

Chappell and Orbach describe Mead's concept of the immediate present as an 'emerging event', by which they mean that the fleeting moment of the present cannot be a precise repetition of what has gone before but is inevitably different from events which are now memories of the past (1986: 84). Memories are connected to the present and the future by 'imagery', for the past is 'remembered and reconstructed from the present' (p. 85). Caro's experience of ageing can never be the same as that of her grandparents, because she is living at a different time and in an ever-changing situation. Nor can she completely identify with the other residents (although she does develop a sympathetic relationship with one bedridden older man) because she cannot occupy their space or live inside their heads. Like all of us, she can understand their problems but is unable to stop being herself. Her ageing is not theirs, or ours (though we may identify sympathetically with her plight and her justified anger), but her own – as imagined, of course, by her author.

By way of illustration Chappell and Orbach (1986) refer to a woman in her seventies, now widowed and her children away from home. She has recently come under the influence of feminist ideas concerning the role of women in society and consequently looks back on her past life as a wife and carer from an altered present. There has, they point out, been no change in her experiences which are part of the past but her interpretation is now different. Viewed through the lens of critical feminism they have taken on a new meaning.

The idea that the present is always elusive helps us to understand the dilemma at the heart of ageing – namely the problem of making sense of the experience of time passing and coming to terms with change. Doris Lessing captures this dilemma very neatly in her novel *Love Again* when she describes Sarah Durham examining herself before a mirror for signs of changes in her appearance that may have taken place over the short period of time covered by the novel. Sarah, a respected professional theatrical director, has fallen in love with Bill, an actor aged 26, and has lived through a series of emotional upheavals. When the novel opens Sarah sees herself as young for her 65 years. She looks at herself approvingly in the mirror and sees 'an apparently middle aged woman' who is energetic, confident, and scarcely concerned about her appearance. After all, she knows she is 'often thought twenty years younger than her real age.' Her body is 'trim' and there is little grey in her hair (Lessing 1996: 6). As the story unfolds and her love affair develops, she consults her reflection more frequently and with a degree of concentrated attention she previously considered unnecessary.

Lessing's novel is about the role that the powerful emotion of love between a younger man and an older woman may play in the process of age consciousness. Although the main focus of the story is on Sarah's increasing self-consciousness of her age identity, other characters too, including the younger men, are aware of time and change. One of the interesting features of the novel is that unlike some other stories about age-discrepant love, there is no sexual interaction. The reader is made aware of Sarah's consciousness of her body and face solely through descriptions of her own perceptions of her appearance in the mirror. Throughout the story Sarah consults her mirror with much greater frequency, we are told, than in the past and this practice is partly seen as gendered. A 'woman's interaction with her mirror', Lessing writes, 'is likely to go through some changes during the decades' (1996: 191). But more generally, interaction with the mirror is represented as the pursuit of the truth of ageing. At one point Lessing sees Sarah's use of the mirror as almost 'scientific' (p. 191), a device for objectively reflecting back to the observer the marks left by the passing of time on the human face and body.

In her pursuit of the truth of ageing, Sarah examines her face and body for two kinds of evidence of the ageing process: external and internal. She looks first of all for any visible signs of change on the surfaces of her face and body. The mirror image holds up pretty well under her scrutiny when she keeps her body still, but when she moves her body 'a subtle disintegration sets in, and areas shapely enough were surfaced with the fine velvety wrinkles of an elderly peach' (Lessing 1996: 234). Second, Sarah looks for signs of the internal changes she imagines have taken place in her body as she has lived her life over the years. These efforts to discover some external record of internal change are expressed as the metaphor of geological upheaval in a landscape. There is for Sarah no escaping the fact that the accumulation of years of past experience 'was like one of those landscapes where subterranean upheavals had tumbled to the surface a dozen strata, each created in vastly different epochs and kept separate until now' (p. 235). This is a vivid image, corresponding in certain respects to the American writer Wendy Chapkis' (1986) picture of the body of the ageing woman as a 'constantly changing landscape' rather than 'a still life of unchanging "perfection"'. The static view, she argues, 'is no praise for creatures so lively and diverse as womankind' (p. 17).

At the end of the story Sarah looks for one last time in the mirror: Months have passed. Sarah is looking into her mirror, just as on the evening when we first saw her. At first glance she has not much changed, but a closer look says otherwise. She has aged by ten years. For one thing, her hair, which for so long remained like a smooth dulled metal, now has grey bands across the front. She has acquired that slow cautious look of the elderly, as if afraid of what they will see around the next corner.

(Lessing 1996: 337)

In this chapter, the body is conceptualized as the fundamental fact of biological existence in which the symbolic elaboration of the self is grounded or embodied. Sarah scrutinizes her body in the mirror to find signs of her subjective experience of changing into what she considers to be an aged self (the reader has no idea whether she is regarded in this light by others, but there is certainly a sense that she has been through a transitional experience and has survived). The body, as I stated earlier, comes first, but from the symbolic interactionist perspective it must always be understood in relation to or in interaction with the self and other people. In the remaining two sections of this chapter we look more closely at the two aspects of body/self consciousness briefly introduced above in the excerpts from Doris Lessing: first, the issue of the external appearance of the ageing body and second, the question of the internal, invisible, body. Here I shall draw heavily on Drew Leder's (1990) concept of the 'dys-appearing body', by which he means the internal body that intrudes into our lives by making us conscious of its presence – as happens, for example in discomfort, or pain (Leder 1990: 69–99).

A troublesome bodily intrusion of the kind Leder has in mind occurs in Alan Isler's *The Prince of West End Avenue* when a group of residents in luxurious residential accommodation in New York put on a performance of Shakespeare's *Hamlet*. Tosca Dawidowicz almost magically transforms herself before the audience from 'an obese, embittered old woman in a gray sweatsuit' into Ophelia, and the spellbinding effect of her performance is 'broken only when the scene came to an end. "My bladder's about to burst! Me first for the little girl's room." The whole company applauded as she ran for the wings' (Isler 1996: 204–5).

When the body 'dys-appears' we may find our present self has become precarious where once perhaps it seemed impregnable. One of the central problems of ageing is the sense of heightened physical vulnerability and risk. In Leder's view we live a great deal of our lives without being fully aware of the internal workings of the body which, when it is free of pain, disability and illness, we experience as 'absent'.

Although we are embodied creatures and therefore cannot live without our bodies, the ideal condition is one where the body only intrudes into our consciousness in pleasurable ways as, for example, when we deliberately look for pleasurable stimulation in food, drink or sex. When we are ill or suffering some of the physical difficulties associated with living a longer life, the body pushes itself into our consciousness or, in Leder's word 'dys-appears' through illness, pain or some sort of dysfunction. 'When reading a book', Leder writes, 'or lost in thought, my own bodily state may be the farthest thing from my awareness. I experientially dwell in a world of ideas, paying little heed to my physical sensations or posture' (1990: 1). But when the body is in pain it makes its presence felt and this is especially the case in the internal organs of the body which are concealed from view. Levels of pain and discomfort can be so intense or prolonged that they blot out everything else from our minds and submerge the self in bodily discomfort. This is the problem which occurs in certain kinds of cancer when the body takes us over and monopolizes all our attention as may happen in a hospice (Lawton 1998).

In the sense in which Leder uses the term much of our life experience is essentially 'disembodied'. A state of health for example is when the body is absent and we are able to forget all about it. The absent body is the body which has, temporarily at least, disappeared from our lives. As we grow chronologically older there is an increasing possibility that the body will appear or 'dys-appear' as pain, discomfort or dysfunction. This influence spreads outwards to the person's immediate social circle. In other words, ageing makes us aware of the body both as an internally functioning system and as the external visible expression of our personal sense of selfhood. In Nina Bawden's *Family Money*, the husband of Fanny's cleaner Ivy has had a stroke. This medical incident not only puts him into hospital but also produces observable changes in his wife's face and the movements of her body. Fanny observes her facial expression and body language: 'How *Ivy* felt was clear to see. She looked devastated; her rosy face pale, her mouth trembling. Her hands shook too much to fasten her seat belt' (Bawden 1997: 116).

Vulnerability is also associated with the exposure of the home to the 'risk invasion' and with the threatening and user-unfriendly nature of public places to older people. As contexts for ageing, places make an enormously supportive contribution to a sense of person security but they can also be full of risk.

External appearance

The most obvious signs of ageing are those visibly displayed on the exposed external surfaces of the face and body. These signs do not usually cause any physical discomfort, nor do they seriously affect our bodily functions. They are therefore largely symbolic, by which I mean they are given an aesthetic or moral significance. In western culture the face has for several centuries been the most exposed part of the body and as such is the designated site of selfhood. In Ann Granger's crime story *Say It With Poison*, Meredith Mitchell visits her actress cousin and contrasts her cousin's portrait painted a few years ago with her face as Meredith now sees it:

> Looking at it, Meredith realised that Eve had changed, only a little, but it was there. The dark tawny-blond hair still looked much as it had in this painting. The fine violet eyes stared out as confidently but in real life the skin beneath them was just starting to sag a little. The jaw line in this picture was firmer. Either the artist had flattered or, again the slight loss of tension of skin and muscle had come over the last year or so. What the artist had done was blatantly ignore the mesh of fine lines which had marked Eve's skin since she had turned thirty, the legacy of hot bright lights, dusty, windswept, sun-drenched locations, heavy stage make-up and the famous wide, beautiful smile which had slowly led to crow's feet in the corners of the eyes and little vertical lines either side of the mouth.
>
> (Granger 1991: 21)

Ageing is frequently recorded by novelists in descriptions of gradual changes in the appearance of the face. Although Eve is not yet in her fifties the contrast between the image of her face in the past and her face as perceived in the living present is a good example of what David Lowenthal describes as 'the look of age' (1986: 125–82). The 'look of age' in this instance is the face which displays signs of experience and the passing of time. However, the 'look of age' also involves perceiving similarities between changes in human appearance, and changes in places and material objects. The look of age is one where many things:

> seem biologically aged owing to erosion or accretion. Ageing is a worn chair, a wrinkled face, a corroded tin, an ivy-covered or mildewed wall; it is a house with sagging eaves, flaking paint, furnishings faded by time and use. Whatever their historical connections, objects that are weathered, decayed, or bear the marks of long-continued use *look* aged and thus seem to stem from the past.
>
> (Lowenthal 1986: 125)

Anna and Ike Robison in Jane Smiley's *At Paradise Gate* have been married for 52 years and Ike, a farmer, is very ill and dependent on Anna, his carer. Formerly a strong authoritarian figure of a man, Ike's face now epitomizes the look of age. Here he is seen through Anna's eyes after he has woken her up during the night: 'He brought his hands down from his face and put them in his lap. Electric light in the middle of the night gave his lips and cheeks an odd clayey color, and brought out the liver spots on his forehead. Though she knew it must be the light, she was taken aback' (Smiley 1995: 94–5).

When in Marika Cobbold's *Guppies For Tea* Amelia calls to collect her confused and troublesome grandmother Selma from Cherryfield retirement home her attention is caught as Selma raises her arms to be dressed by the nurse. She 'stared at the bones that seemed like a giant clothes hanger holding up the sagging flesh. She glanced at her own arms, bare in a short-sleeved T-shirt, as if making sure of their firm roundness and the honey-tone of the skin before turning away guiltily' (Cobbold 1993: 149). Amelia's affection for her grandmother almost knows no bounds but she cannot prevent herself from a surreptitious act of invidious comparison between Selma's body and her own in confirmation of her comparative youth.

The 'look of age' in human beings is, generally speaking, considered unwelcome and undesirable. Old buildings and objects showing signs of wear and tear may well be evaluated highly as 'antiques' or 'collectibles', but in western culture the people most likely to be aesethetically and morally celebrated are those who do not 'look their age' (Hepworth and Featherstone 1982). For a number of reasons (Elias 1985) the visual appearance of the ageing face and body is unsettling both for ourselves and others, and until very recently the naked body was regarded in western art as unaesthetic unless idealistically represented (Kent 1991). And change in this respect is very gradual and uneven. When in Minette Walters' *The Scold's Bridle* it is discovered that the older woman who is the murder victim had been painted in the nude by Jack, a young artist, the reaction is one of suspicion and unease. After all, older women do not normally expose their bodies in this way. To do so even in contemporary society is to deliberately challenge and provoke:

> Joanna turned back to her with a frown. 'I suppose you know she posed in the nude for him. I found one of his sketches in her desk. It left nothing

to the imagination, I can assure you. Do you call that dignified? She was old enough to be his mother.'

'It depends on your point of view. If you regard the female nude as intrinsically demeaning or deliberately provocative, then, yes, I suppose you could say it was undignified of Mathilda.' She shrugged. 'But that's a dangerous philosophy which belongs to the dark ages and more intolerant religions. . . . If, on the other hand you see the nude figure, be it male or female, as one of nature's creations, and therefore as beautiful and as extraordinary as anything else on this planet, then I see no shame involved in allowing a painter to paint it.'

(Walters 1995: 169)

The discussion in the above conversation is, of course, about the moral and asethetic significance of the ageing body. The external appearance of biological ageing when not interfered with cosmetically is a fact of life but the meanings we attribute to this fact are variable. It is still largely the case, however, that the ageing body is more acceptable (sexually and otherwise) the closer it approximates to youth. Like Sarah Durham before she came to believe her experiences of love had aged her (Lessing 1996), we all gratefully welcome any physical signs that we may be wearing better than those around us. Thus Simon Brett's Mrs Pargeter, in *Mrs Pargeter's Package*, a wealthy and rumbustious wealthy widow in her sixties:

moved a little further down the beach, took a towel out of her bag and laid it down on the stones. Then she slipped off the cotton dress to reveal a brightly printed bikini beneath. Hers was more substantial than those worn by the two secretaries, but made no attempt to hide her voluptuousness. Mrs Pargeter knew her skin to be smooth and unmarked, and people who found plumpness unattractive were under no obligation to look at her. 'My Goddess of Plenty', that was how the late Mr Pargeter had always referred to her, she remembered fondly as she stepped in sandalled feet down to the sea.

(Brett 1992a: 86)

And in Robert Barnard's crime story *Posthumous Papers*, the second Mrs Machin is described in terms of her contrived display of the traces of a former youthful sexual allure:

. . . she was substantial, imposing, must even in her time have been voluptuous. Her clothes announced emphatically that they were not chain-store products: a full beige cape swirled abundantly round her full figure and was topped by a simple pudding-basin hat of brown velvet, with a massive shady brim. She was a model of style for the elderly, and to complete the picture she had on a bright red lead a sprightly black poodle. In earlier days . . . she would have sailed forward with the splendid confidence of a fine woman. Now she seemed to have trouble with her ankles, and she walked carefully, seeming all the time to be chafing against her carefulness.

(Barnard 1992: 8)

It seems, therefore, that it is very difficult (at least in our western culture at the present time) to construct positive images of the external appearance of the ageing body without some reference to comparative moral and aesthetic evaluations of youth and age. The look of age is always symbolically elaborated in terms of its opposite, the 'look of youth'. Thus, for example, in Kingsley Amis' *The Biographer's Moustache*, after Gordon Scott-Thompson, a young writer has gone to bed with an older woman, Joanna Fane, he gets a glimpse of her naked back when she leaves the room. This view of her body is 'not quite as good as he would perhaps have liked but good enough to lend some support to the belief he had more than once heard expressed, that of ladies of more mature years the part below the neck retained the look of youth longer than that above' (Amis 1996: 118).

As the example from Amis implies, the look of youth is for biological reasons difficult to retain across the entire surface of the body and is often visibly displayed only in selected parts. Parts of the body can take on a special symbolic significance when they are seen as 'standing in' for an entire self. Teeth have an interesting role as a visible symbol of the ageing self. In her analysis of 'contemporary midlife fiction', Margaret Gullette has observed that the central characters often 'start having trouble with their teeth'. She cites Saul Bellow's novel *Henderson the Rain King*, where Eugene Henderson breaks one of the bridges on his teeth biting on a hard biscuit and experiences feelings of anger, fear, and disgust: 'there were tears in my eyes' (Gullette 1988: 1). Citing the belief that teeth are a symbol of both wisdom and sexual vigour, Gullette shows how broken teeth, lost fillings and dentures are seen as indicative of an ageing self. Teeth problems in mid-life can be interpreted as the sign of the onset of decline.

A perfect row of teeth has of course been of increasing importance as the smile has become an increasingly valued sign of the socially acceptable self. Less than perfect teeth can be a problem as John Woodforde (1983) noted in his history of false teeth. The absence of teeth is a source of low social status and personal worth resulting in feelings of disgust and revulsion. Woodforde suggests that it was in Britain in the 1920s when writers began to use false teeth to indicate 'character'. 'It became', he writes, 'almost a convention that insecure or troublesome ones make a suitable attribute for a person who is himself in some way insecure' (1983: 123). In 'H.E. Bates' touching story *The Major of Hussars*, a double set of teeth, cherished and gleaming but inclined to slip, comes between an elderly man and his far-too-young wife. The story ends with an overheard bedroom scene in which the young woman 'hurls the teeth against a wall.' (Woodforde 1983: 123).

Like many of the material signs of selfhood, and especially ageing selfhood, false teeth are open to critical scrutiny and evaluation. The reactions of embarrassment and disgust they may induce are related to their symbolic function of displaying a physically intact self. Missing and broken teeth in stories of ageing are frequently compared with symbols of death. Amelia, the young central character in Marika Cobbold's *Guppies For Tea*, is sitting in a train opposite an old man when they pass a large graveyard. Amelia is immediately reminded of 'giant teeth, or old crumbling white, streaked by years of rain like powdered cheeks' (Cobbold 1993: 51). She looks over at the man and wonders what his reaction is to this image of death: ' "Nice day," smiled the old man, showing a perfect set of white dentures' (p. 52).

As artificial aids to mastication and self-presentation the social and personal acceptability of false teeth increases in direct proportion to the skill with which they are imbued with a 'natural' quality. To be artificially 'natural' implies a closer merging of the ageing body with the look of youth, which is why the manipulation of false teeth accentuates the appearance of age even when done playfully, as in an incident in Jane Smiley's *At Paradise Gate* when, during a conversation with his children and grandchildren about a 'sweet tooth' for caramels, 'Ike dislodged his false teeth and pushed them out of his mouth in a picket-fence grin, then drew them back in again' (Smiley 1995: 30).

If the teeth can be seen as symbols of the self, the eyes have even greater significance as images of our subjective inner lives. Eyes, in western think-ing, play a dual role. They are considered to be our foremost source of in-formation about the external world and also the 'windows of the soul' or essential self (Jay 1994; Kern 1996). In Celia Dale's *A Helping Hand*, part of Josh Evans' presentation of a caring self when he sets out to con the widowed Cynthia Fingal out of her money is not only his 'smiling attention' but his 'kind eyes' (Dale 1990b: 22–3).

When a person is seriously ill in later life and physically restricted, the eyes may be accentuated by a writer to emphasize either an inner strength or the signs of a vigorous character in the past. In *Kill the Lights*, Simon Williams gives a good example of this in an encounter between Dominic and Lady Charlotte, who is suffering from Parkinson's disease:

> Her whole body was shaking to some gentle motor out of sight. Only in her eyes was there any stillness. 'Don't worry about strange sp . . . sp . . . speaking voice. Horrid, yes?' Her mouth jerked into a smile as she waved him to a wing chair. She fumbled with the remote control and stabbed the television to silence. Her disease was like a quicksand she told him.
>
> (Williams 1993: 292)

A similar example from a first encounter between a younger and an older person occurs in P.D. James' *A Taste for Death* when her detective, Comman-der Adam Dalgliesh, comes into the presence of the invalid Lady Ursula. It is her eyes that draw his attention. They are, he observes, 'still remarkable, immense, well-spaced and heavily lidded. They must once have been the focus of her beauty, and although they were sunken now, he could still see the glint of intelligence behind them' (James 1986: 100–1). The past self of Lady Ursula had been beautiful and intelligent. As a younger woman Lady Charlotte in Simon Williams' novel had been Dominic's father's mistress and she is described as surrounded by photographs showing her 'in her middle years, always in a headscarf or a hat – a kind face that was probably more beautiful in repose' (Williams 1993: 290).

All these examples point to the wider issue involving all of us as we grow older: namely, the problem of symbolically expressing our sense of continuous inner selfhood through the biologically changing body. Because novels are concerned with identifiable individuals, fictional descriptions of the physical processes of human ageing are always used to indicate characteristics of the self and the same is true in social life. Bryan Turner (1995) has noted how the sociologist Norbert Elias, in his book *The Loneliness of the Dying* (1985), written in his mid-eighties, spoke of ageing 'precisely in terms of the physical trans-formation of his *own* body. The passage of time is experientially measured by the passing of *his* body'. We need, says Turner, to continuously 'remind our-selves always of the centrality of our bodies to experience' (1995: 250). We can't speak of memories of the past without referring to the remembered body in the past. Hillel Schwartz (1989) put the same issue slightly differently when he said that human beings have three bodies: the body in the past, the body in the present, and the body in the future.

In the majority of examples cited so far it is the perspective of the outside observer that has been the most prominent. One exception has been Doris Lessing's Sarah Durham in *Love Again* who we saw examining her face and body in the mirror for signs of correspondence between her ageing body and her ageing self. I shall now close this section of the discussion of the external appearance of the face and body with some further thoughts on the question of mirrors.

Examples of older people looking in mirrors for signs of ageing are com-monplace. The mirror is now an indispensable aid to body and self-examin-ation. In Julian Rathbone's *Blame Hitler*, Thomas Somers, aged 59, goes into the bathroom and looks at himself in the full-length mirror 'as if he were a doctor with a new patient'. His self-examination is not, however, as clinical and objective as the medical metaphor implies because his inventory of bodily strengths and weaknesses is personalized. The body he sees reflected in the mirror is *his* body but also in certain respects a family body. He notices 'his left foot had a bunion' which is not simply a medical condition but is 'just like his mother's' (Rathbone 1998: 74); he takes note of the bags under his eyes, drawing comfort from their genealogy: 'those bags go back at least as far as great-grandad Philip Henry Somers', and his nose is not so bulbous as was his father's (p. 75). Somers is particularly preoccupied with physical signs of ageing because when he reaches the age of 60 he will be older than his father when he died and is seriously troubled by thoughts that he is not morally worthy to live longer. His comparative inventory is part of his wider concern with ageing as a moral process where the self is in close symbolic interaction with others now dead.

This example suggests that the mirror is not a device for discovering the objective truth about the body but a surface on which we perceive reflected images of the way we imagine that others see us. In symbolic interactionist terms we construct a 'looking-glass self': the 'I' is perceived in relation to the 'me' and is constructed symbolically out of the ways that 'I' imagine I appear to others. In Stanley Middleton's *Necessary Ends* Sam Martin, retired and in his eighties, is attracted to Alice Jeffreys who is 20 years younger. He exam-ines his face in the mirror and sees it as 'blotched, marred, mole-ugly, lacking grace and symmetry'. On the positive side he can read 'character' and 'experi-ence' in his features but on the negative side he fears that he lacks the 'beauty' he imagines Alice will require to 'attract' and 'dazzle her' (Middleton 1999: 107).

Although we can extend our visual access to the external appearance of our own bodies through the use of mirrors and other technical aids including photographic and other images, these perspectives are never objective abstractions without symbolic meaning. When we look into a mirror we do not get a direct sight of our own body and self; we see ourselves as others see us. In Henry Sutton's *Gorleston*, Percy the retired widower goes out shopping to buy clothes. His self-consciousness has been changed by his infatuation with Queenie, a lively and sexually provocative older woman. Percy wishes to impress Queenie so when he looks in the mirror he is really wondering how he will appear in *her* eyes:

> He wanted to feel and look rather decadent. Standing by the rack he took his jacket off and put on a silk burgundy dressing gown over his pullover. . . . He imagined walking through his home, out into the garden on a summer's morning, with his thin legs looking whiter than ever against the dark red hue. . . .
> 'That's the right choice.'
> He knew the voice instantly.
> 'Looks great. Who's the lucky lady?'
>
> (Sutton 1995: 77–8)

In *Passing On* by Penelope Lively Helen, an unmarried woman aged 52 is attracted to Giles Carnaby, her solicitor. But in her head she hears her deceased mother's voice continually reminding her that there is no chance of the relationship developing because she has never been a beauty and she should try 'to pull herself together and think about something else' (Lively 1989: 53). She arrives home, takes off all her clothes and inspects her body closely in a long mirror and sees, as she imagines through the eyes of her mother and Carnaby, a body that is unlikely to hold out any attractions. At this moment her own age consciousness emerges out of a symbolic interaction between her mirror image and her ability to adopt what she imagines to be the attitudes of others towards what she can see. Helen makes a deliberate effort to look into the mirror to try to discover the truth about herself. The truth she is looking for is in the final analysis the product of her imagination, if only because the other people whose opinion is influential (her mother and Giles Carnaby) have never seen her naked body as it now is.

If we don't care what others think we may have fewer problems with our appearance: in Margaret Forster's *The Seduction of Mrs Pendlebury*, Mrs Pendlebury, who is a much older woman than Helen, looks at her face in the mirror and 'touched her hair and pinched her white sagging cheeks. She looked terrible, but there was no one but herself to tell her that she looked terrible and she did not take much notice of herself' (Forster 1978: 12). It is not that Mrs Pendlebury's husband, like Helen's mother, is dead, or that she lives alone, but simply that she is not concerned about her husband's opinion.

For Hollander (1988) the image we see in the mirror is 'the personal link between the human subject and its representation' (p. 391). Far from being engaged in the objective perception of the body and self, 'the mirror gazer is engaged in creating a posed studio portrait of himself, not even a candid shot . . . the mirror viewer must . . . always watch himself looking at himself. . . .

The very act of consulting the mirror presupposes some will to create an image, to fill the frame deliberately' (pp. 392–3).

Looking into the mirror is an interactive process through which connections are made between the personal subjective self of the viewer and the external world of other people. Because we have no direct access to the external reality of the body, even with the assistance of aids such as mirrors and the wide range of technical apparatus now available (cameras, video cameras and the like), the act of human perception is always mediated symbolically by meaning. When we look into a mirror we are therefore engaged in an act of the imagination whereby the self is constructed symbolically as a portrait or picture.

The construction of the self as a picture extends, of course, from the appearance of the face as a symbol of the self to include the external appearance of the body as we imagine it looks to other people. In western culture, the 'normal' body (and in particular the ageing body) is the clothed as distinct from the naked body and dress, as Percy out shopping in the novel *Gorleston* (Sutton 1995) discovered, can be seen as 'an integral part of the self' (Hollander 1988: 424). In this respect we never see the body entirely naked but always in relation to items of clothing we have temporarily discarded or rearranged – what Hollander describes as 'the personal dressed self' (1988: 391).

The 'dys-appearing body'

The visual appearance of the visible face and the body exercises a crucial influence over the emergence of the self from infancy, and we gradually develop self-consciousness as we become aware of the interpretations other people make of our appearance. But although we are exposed to constant reminders about our external appearance, even if these are only partial views of our own bodies and inevitably mediated by the perceptions of others, our knowledge of the internal workings of the body is even more limited.

As we noted earlier in this chapter, Drew Leder describes the problem of the inner body as the 'dys-appearing body' by which he means the body that makes its presence felt as pain, disease and dysfunction (1990: 69–99). To give another fictitious example of what he means, in Deborah Moggach's *Close Relations*, Gordon Hammond at the age of 65 has an unexpected heart attack. As a result he goes into hospital where his body is 'taken away from him', handed over to a series of professionals who turn him into a medical case history to be probed, prodded and manipulated into recovery. Gordon's dys-appearing body is described as follows:

> Only the pain belonged to him but even that seemed like an unwelcome visitor, an intruder that had lodged in his chest and stolen his normal sensations. It dared him to shift his position. It lurked, heavy and serious, beneath his ribcage and lingered in his leg where the angioplasty had been pushed into his vein. Over the past two days alien instruments had intimately explored his body; they were accompanied by a technical vocabulary with which he was now becoming familiar, though it still gave him a jolt when he realised that it was applied to himself.
>
> (Moggach 1997: 103)

The heart attack has temporarily transformed Gordon from person to 'patient' or body. He experiences the pain and the medical treatment as distanced from the self he has created over the years in his work as a successful self-employed builder, happily married husband, and father of grown-up children. Until this medical episode, Gordon has managed to ignore his body and to regard it as 'absent' (Leder 1990).

Leder's main argument is that although we are essentially biological creatures we live, especially in relatively affluent societies where basic physical needs are satisfied, as though the body does not exist (is 'absent'). That is to say, in its ideal form we prefer the body to leave us alone to get on with our lives. We are, of course, constantly reminded that we have bodies (women more than men because of the nature of their reproductive function) but these reminders are comparatively mild in their intensity and duration. We know we have to eat, to digest food, to excrete waste products but we try to live our lives in such a way that the potential of such functions for disrupting our lives is under control. Alternatively, we stimulate the body into consciousness in pleasurable ways through the cultivation of the 'natural' appetites.

The 'dys-appearing body' makes its presence felt in unpleasant and, as in Gordon's case, life-threatening ways. Mrs Parminter, in Kathleen Rowntree's *Mr Brightly's Evening Off*, is out in her garden one day when she becomes aware she has been lying in the rose bed for some period of time. She does not know how long. Having come round from this sudden lapse in consciousness she has to manoeuvre the body she had far less trouble getting into the garden out of its supine position from the rose bed and back into the house. Mrs Parminter's body, the 'absent' agent of her selfhood, has become 'the body', a cumbersome and unwieldy object to be manipulated with as much ingenuity as she can muster:

> She rehearsed what she must do: onto her hands and knees she must go; and therefore, because her left knee and hip were swollen with arthritis, her right knee must come over to take the strain, to act as a lever against the ground. With a great heave she thrust over: only to discover that she had neglected to take into account the proximity of the Lili Marlene. She shuffled her bottom closer to the Ballerina and tried again.
>
> (Rowntree 1997: 14)

Mrs Parminter's body has not, of course, been entirely absent because as an older woman she suffers from arthritis, but the point is that other internal changes associated with ageing have been taking place below her level of consciousness.

Because a great deal of the complex and variable process of physical ageing does not take place on the visible surfaces of the body it is not surprising that we may 'suddenly' become aware that we are ageing. As Kathleen Woodward has noted, 'history and its time, is written not only on the body but *inside* the body. Opening up the body in age, then, may represent *seeing* the disturbing disjunction between the chronological age of the body (the organs of the body "speak" the age of the person and its (soon to be) remodelled outside' (1991: 164–5). The fact that the depths of the internal body are usually concealed from us – that there are 'vast gaps in our inner perception' – means that 'potentially damaging processes' may be concealed until they are 'far advanced' (Thompson *et al.* 1990: 43). When someone says 'I don't feel old', he or she is describing the body as non-intrusive or absent. It is for this reason that ageing is difficult to imagine when we are comparatively young. In his opening remarks to a lecture he gave to a medical conference in 1983, Norbert Elias, in his eighties, made a poignant comparison between the difference in imagining one is old when one is young and actually experiencing the ageing body in later life. By way of illustration he recalled an incident from the past:

> An experience I had in my younger days has taken on a certain signifi-cance for me, now that I am older. I attended a lecture by a well-known physicist at Cambridge. He came in shuffling, dragging his feet, a very old man. I caught myself wondering, Why does he drag his feet like that? Why can he not walk like a normal human being? I at once corrected myself. He can't help it, I told myself. He is very old.
>
> (Elias 1985: 68)

Elias had, as he grew older, discovered that old age as imagined when we are young is not quite the same thing as the direct experience of 'how it feels when muscle tissue gradually hardens and perhaps becomes fatty, when con-nective tissue multiplies and cell renewal slows down' (1985: 69).

In Leder's (1990) view the intrusion of the 'dys-appearing body' helps to explain why there are times when we experience the self as existing separ-ately from the body. When the body functions smoothly and without pain or discomfort we experience body and self in terms of harmonious performance. When the body is absent it is much easier to believe in the unity of self and body but, when the smooth functioning of the body is interrupted in some way and begins to bother us, the self may appear to become detached from the body and we may imagine we are disembodied creatures. Because the body is fortunately so often absent, marginally intrusive or pleasurably stimu-lated, it seems as if it the body has nothing to do with the self. The 'dys-appearing body' leads to the belief that self and the body have a separate existence. In addition, the human capacity for symbolization also encourages us to detach the self from the body. The human ability to manipulate symbols to give the body meaning also creates the impression that the self can be lib-erated from the body and can persist in a disembodied form. But when the body seriously makes its presence felt, the self we felt so comfortable with can be blurred or undermined. In pain, the body appears as an 'alien presence' (Leder 1990: 76) and a cleavage is experienced between the body and the self as we become more preoccupied with our bodies. The 'old' self 'dys-appears'. In Jane Smiley's *At Paradise Gate*, Anna, aged 72 and caring for Ike, aged 77, writes to her cousin: 'I should have written sooner, but Daddy got sick in Feb-ruary again, and I have my hands full. It is his heart mainly, but I think he is better than he seems, and perhaps as the Spring wears on he will return to his old self' (Smiley 1995: 74).

It is important to stress that ageing and disease, in Leder's view, are not necessarily the same. Ageing is a 'normal and necessary part of the life cycle' and should not be 'associated with the notions of "bad" or "ill" that comprise part of the Greek meaning of *dys'* (1990: 89). Nevertheless the 'ageing person has to adjust to a multitude of physical changes' (1990: 90) and these may well include painful illness and physical deterioration. Ageing can be one of the times in which 'one develops a new closeness to and evaluation of one's body' (1990: 90).

In *Beginning to End*, Stanley Middleton describes the following exchange between an older man, Stapleton, and a younger, Clark. Throughout, Stapleton is described as physically frail and as resentful of his aches and pains:

> 'You've plenty of time. No, I don't mean hours of the day. Years to come. I'm seventy-five, nearly seventy-six. I can't guarantee myself anything. Now you'd think that would have it advantages. For instance, when I walk out into the garden on a fine morning, you would claim that I ought to make the best of it. The sun's shining; I've only myself to please; I'm feeling fit and sprightly. *Carpe diem*. But it's not so.'
>
> 'Why is that, then?'
>
> 'I never feel really well; that's the top and bottom of it. Some bit or piece is aching or creaking. It's not so much death as life that's making a fool of me.'
>
> (Middleton 1991: 31–2)

Later in the novel Stapleton says angrily:

> '. . . The whole of my life consists now of wasting time.'
>
> 'Whose fault is that?
>
> 'Fault? Fault?' Stapleton's voice cracked angrily. 'I'm slow for a start. It takes me half an hour to do a five-minute job. And it's painful. Arthritis, bronchitis and angina do not make a good combination. I was energetic, and hard-working and enterprising. I was a decent solicitor, and I made a lot of money in property.'
>
> (Middleton 1991: 55–6)

3

Self and others

Others as mirrors

The mirror, as we have seen, plays an important part in fostering age consciousness and shaping age identity. But we have noted that it can only
perform this function because we see the reflected image of our face and body
through the ways in which we imagine others see us. As the conversation
between Stapleton and Clark (Middleton 1991) which closed the last chapter
suggests, each individual constructs his or her own version of age identity
from the expectations of others.

In *Intimacy* by Julian Rathbone, Querubin, the ageing castrato master of
baroque singing, prepares to meet his new pupil, a young woman called Petra,
for the first time. He examines his image in the mirror and although his sight
is failing he knows what she will see when they meet:

> Short white hair, an open lightly tanned face, more lined than his sixty-
> nine years would lead you to expect, just a touch oriental around baggy
> eyelids, a body succumbing prematurely to old age, arms thin and a little
> saggy, the torso heavy, the barrel chest that had given his voice such
> power falling away from the prominent breast-bone, and a loose-skinned
> stomach.
>
> (Rathbone 1995: 27)

As a person who has retired from a highly successful career as a performing
artist, Querubin has considerable social and cultural power, and unlike
Thomas Somers in Rathbone's *Blame Hitler* there is no question of any sexual
attraction between the younger woman and the older man, but he is still concerned about the appearance of ageing and its possible negative influence on
the way his new pupil will see him. In both Thomas Somers and Querubin's
eyes the appearance of ageing is seen as a potential stigma in relationships

with younger people. Not everyone, however, is necessarily unhappy with their appearance or the social judgement that they imagine it will provoke. A stereotypical appearance of ageing may be manipulated and exploited to advantage, as in the case of Agatha Christie's Miss Marple.

On the personal or subjective level, age awareness is, therefore, the realization that the self is not fixed for ever, sealed inside us as in an invulnerable body, but a fluid and changing process, dependent on other people and co-extensive with our relationships, the places where we live and the material objects we possess. In other words, the self is part of others.

During her research in the USA into the experience of old age Sharon Kaufman (1986) held up a hand mirror to Millie's face. Millie had suffered a stroke and had been admitted to a nursing home after treatment in hospital. She was asked to look in the glass and describe her image: 'What do you see?' (p. 193). Millie replied 'I go by what people tell me. They say I look 100 percent better than I did. I have changed considerably from what I looked like when I first came here, and I see a more pleasant expression in my face, and I'm more inspired about my routine. . . '. Kaufman adds that 'Millie's reference point for her self-description is other people's remarks about her improved morale and appearance since entering the institution' (p. 152). Millie's self-esteem is enhanced through her awareness of the approval of others.

Age identity and interaction

One of the besetting problems of later life – the ageism issue – is that the kind of approval Millie received is not always available and may be withheld. The stigma of physical ageing may effectively mask the individual self and result in the perpetuation of collective stereotypes. In *A Few Green Leaves*, Barbara Pym describes this process in Dr Martin Shrubshole's attitude to older patients. Dr Shrubshole is the young village doctor with a keen interest in geriatric medicine. He is, however, only interested in older people as medical cases and shies away from any personal involvement with them:

> Although he was a kind man and keenly interested in the elderly and those in late middle age, his interest was detached and clinical. He enjoyed taking blood pressure – even felt an urge to pursue the group of elderly ladies round the rector with his sphygmometer – but was disinclined to enter into other aspects of their lives.
>
> (Pym 1980: 5)

Dr Shrubshole's clinical view of ageing extends to the stereotypically prescriptive and a denial of a fully social self, reflected in his belief that 'the drugs prescribed to control high blood pressure should also damp down emotional excesses and those fires of youth that could still – regrettably – burn in the dried up hearts of those approaching old age' (p. 5).

The denial of full selfhood is the central theme in Anthony Gilbert's crime story *The Spinster's Secret*, where the key events of the story take place in the last months in the life of Miss Janet Martin, the spinster of the title, who has devoted the best years of her life to looking after a 'comfortable invalid' mother (Gilbert 1987: 7). She has reached the age of 74 and suffers from some of the physical frailties and social losses of old age, but is mentally sound. She has weak eyes, receives few letters, and is without relatives except for a niece who she sees occasionally and a well-off married nephew who lives in the North and has 'no time for the unsuccessful' (p. 2). Miss Martin passes the day enjoyably observing the social scene from the window of her bedsitting room in Blakely House. Blakely House offers privately rented sheltered accommodation presided over by the formidable Miss Fraser who believes in adopting a 'brisk' manner towards old ladies who otherwise 'yielded to self-pity, and everyone knew that was fatal' (p. 3). The threat of expulsion, therefore, is an ever-present sanction.

Miss Martin's other enjoyment is derived from going out into the streets observing the activities of those around her and this, of course, is how she discovers her 'secret'. In the first part of the story, Miss Martin's discovery and her attempts to persuade others that a murder has been committed are seen through her own eyes. The reader is invited to share Miss Martin's perception of a truth to which others are blind because they perceive her to be simply another old woman who has become weak in the head and is suffering from delusions. In this respect readers are invited to take sides in Miss Martin's struggle against an unreasoning and socially restrictive stereotype. All her efforts to communicate her suspicions are received unsympathetically and merely confirm the beliefs of those around her, including professional carers, that she is 'taking leave of her senses'. Already perceived as 'odd' by her middle-aged niece, she is removed from Blakely House and admitted to Beverley, 'advertised as a Rest-Home for old ladies requiring light attention and care' (Gilbert 1987: 25).

At Beverley she is forced into unwelcome and close contact with residents who in contrast are conventionally 'dessicated' and confused older women. At tea 'she met her room-mate, a distinctly eccentric old lady, who enlivened the nights by suddenly starting up and crying that they must get ready, for the day of the Lord was at hand, and asking Miss Martin if she too could not see signs and portents in the sky' (Gilbert 1987: 28). As readers are fully aware, Miss Martin's problem is that those who 'care' for her are prevented by their stereotyped theories of old age from recognizing the truth of her claims and distinguishing her from other older people whose perceptions are more clouded and fanciful.

When, in her increasingly urgent attempts to confirm her suspicions and to demonstrate the reality of her claims, she attempts to secretly observe what she believes to be the scene of the murder (a place which appears to others to be an innocent and commonplace domestic residence), she is in turn observed by a doctor's wife who lives in the house opposite:

'What on earth is she doing there?' she wondered, and then she recognised her as the old body who had been hanging around pretending to admire her garden not long before. Curiosity kept her where she was, though she had the sense to pull a curtain forward a little to conceal her presence if the old thing should look up. The old thing, however, behaved as though there was no such building as the house opposite. When the door of the orphanage opened and the two ladies came out she strained even closer to the wall, and it would have been obvious to an idiot that she was eavesdropping. After the car had driven away she came through the gate, obviously quite unaware of the daft appearance she presented, with bits of twigs in her hair and her hat askew, and she went pattering down the road at a great rate.

(Gilbert 1987: 73)

The reader is privileged, of course, because she or he has access to two perspectives: the view from Miss Martin and the alternative interpretation of others. As noted, the story opens with the view from Miss Martin and with the promise (since this is a story about a mysterious crime) that Miss Martin will be vindicated. As an exceptional old lady (she is the only older character in the book who is not 'dessicated' or senile) she is at once a testimony to the power of the traditional stigma of old age (the view from the outside) and evidence of the distorted perceptions of 'reality' that the stigma can produce. Her persistent attempts to uncover evidence to substantiate her suspicions are perceived by the younger characters in the novel as cumulative evidence of her age-induced anti-social eccentricity: ' "I must say", acknowledged Doreen brutally, "she does sound as if she was suffering from brain-softening. Oh, dear! Why can't these old people die off when they're no longer any use to themselves or anyone else?" ' (Gilbert 1987: 116).

The doctor who professionally examines Miss Martin after his wife has informed him that she saw Miss Martin lurking eccentrically in the bushes of the house opposite shares this popular theory of old age:

It was his experience that a good many elderly people became queer, and the best place for senile cases was the institution, unless there was some convenient relative. From what the matron had told him, he was prepared to find Miss Martin peculiar and sign her up, in which case there would be little difficulty in getting his opinion confirmed by another local doctor.

(Gilbert 1987: 116–17)

Fiction is able to show us how our conception of another person's self and its influence over our social dealings is determined by the information available to us and any preconceptions we may hold. Novels are a rich source of information about the tensions between social stereotypes of ageing and the struggle of older individuals to maintain an independent identity as thinking, self-regulating people. In other words, to be credited with a full social self and individual self.

The Spinster's Secret is, therefore, an interesting example of the process of 'holding on to the self and resisting the claims of others' which Anthony Cohen argues is the core issue in the process of ageing into old age. In Cohen's view accounts of the experience of ageing (he is referring to non-fictional accounts but the argument can be extended to apply to fiction) 'all lead to the conclusion that the reassertion of selfhood against its social subversion is an essential element in the life work of the elderly' (1994: 99). This argument is also central to Kitwood's (1998) analysis of the negative consequences of denying selfhood, or 'personhood' as he prefers to call it, to individuals who are suffering from Alzheimer's disease. In his view when 'persons-with-dementia' begin to experience difficulties in expressing the self it is the responsibility of carers to maintain that self through social interaction. The self thus passes from the individual back to the group.

Fiction allows, as we have seen, the reader to participate in sequences of social interaction from a number of perspectives. This is particularly the case in stories of ageing in Variations 1 and 2 outlined in Chapter 1. We see not only the visible outward surface appearance of people but are given privileged insight into their mental processes and perceptions of situations, and their motivations. In *A View of the Harbour*, Elizabeth Taylor's Mrs Bracey is paralysed from the hip down and confined to her bed. She allows her mind to range freely over life in the form of an inner conversation and enjoys embarrassing her daughter with bawdy and irreverent observations. For many in the harbour town she is merely a 'prying old gossip with a very spiteful tongue' (Taylor 1995: 263), but Bernard Hemingway, a retired man, a stranger, spends some time with her at her bedside when she is dying, and sees her as a person with unrealized potential whose ability to express her talents has been narrowly restricted by gender, social class and ill-health. In the passages describing the interaction between the two of them we are given a glimpse of a person of greater complexity than the bawdy and embarrassing gossip. In this character study of an older bedridden woman the novelist shows us that no one is as simple as they outwardly appear.

In *Guppies For Tea* by Marika Cobbold, we see into the mind of the confused Selma who is in bed and waiting for her husband we know is dead to join her, and thus for a moment we are able to imagine her state of mind and to appreciate her confusion. Another good example of fiction as an imaginative resource is the dementing Serena Burley in Frances Hegarty's *Let's Dance*, where we enter Serena's own mind as she struggles to write down her confused thoughts in her journal during the early hours of the morning. And we see how Serena interacts in her imagination with her journal, with photographs and with the voices she hears. We see her through the eyes of her daughter Isabel, who sets her own life aside to look after her mother in the large family home in the depths of the country. We also see Serena from the perspective of the psychiatric nurse who Isabel consults. The nurse offers a cheerfully detached clinical perspective on dementia which turns Serena into an interesting case history: ' "Lessened ability to perform ordinary domestic tasks, rather more eccentric about appearance, less physical coordination. Suffers slightly from persecution mania, which I don't remember noting before. Claims to have been bludgeoned by the cat" ' (Hegarty 1996: 204).

Isabel, however, finds this less than satisfactory because she has to live with Serena not as a clinical category but as a person, and she feels the strains on herself as carer are being ignored or blithely sidelined. The novel therefore gives us glimpses of Isabel's resentment when her mother becomes difficult and when she roams around the house in the early hours of the morning and disturbs her sleep:

> she couldn't cope, not without sleep. Mother, please do not be an inconsiderate old bitch. The phrase, fully formed, popped into her mind, anger

getting her out of bed with such speed she made herself dizzy, and angered herself more. She would throw that tape deck and radio out of the house, she would too. Start wearing earplugs, scream.

(Hegarty 1996: 173)

Older people are not necessarily transformed or made any easier by physical dependency, and the interaction between carer and cared-for can impose restrictions on the carer's self expression. In *Let's Dance*, Frances Hegarty describes the relationship between Andrew Cornell, who is an unmarried male carer, and his father as follows:

Andrew had spent almost eight years of his life nursing his father after a car smash which had never curtailed his drinking or dulled the old man's wits. Doc Reilly said that this was how the boy had learned his love of a good antique. Both of them had resented it. John was not made kinder by disablement and the youthful Andrew had been poised for flight, which now felt too late for the prematurely middle-aged man he had become.

(Hegarty 1996: 37)

As this passage shows, Andrew has not entirely lost out in this relationship because he has become skilled in his father's business and has prospered materially. The price, however, has been his loss of youth and a corresponding personal sense of being prematurely aged.

The complex pressures of caring for an old and ailing husband are sensitively and sympathetically detailed in Jane Smiley's *At Paradise Gate*. Anna, caring for her husband, looks at the sleeping Ike and ponders the sense of resentment she experiences. She has been faithful to Ike for 52 years and now he has become ill she cares for him diligently, and yet:

Why did she fail to rise to the occasion of this illness every day? Why did she meet every demand with resentment and reluctance, or take refuge all the time in gardening plans or sewing plans, or lately, fruitless reminiscing? . . . Obviously he was very sick and getting sicker, and she acted as if he were merely perverse. She thought of him dead, right now dead in the unspeaking bulk of the dark house. . . .

(Smiley 1995: 108–9)

This example exposes the reflexive influence of the caring relationship on the self-consciousness of the carer, on her personal awareness of ageing. One feature of Anna's age identity is the conflicting pressures of a sense of domestic duty and personal desire for self-fulfilment. At one point in Smiley's narrative Anna is provoked into pushing Ike, now physically weak, with some force into his chair – an action which indicates a shift in the balance of power between the once physical, powerful and dominant male and the subservient, caring wife. Caring is not only a matter of bearing the 'burden' of the immediate practical tasks to hand but also a matter of working reflexively through the life review such duties provoke. In the course of ministering to Ike and her family Anna experiences at one point in the story a deep sense of anger over a lifetime of caring: 'she had not stopped feeding . . . for half a century.

She was furious. She had to go to bed. Why did they treat her house, her larder, her furniture, her effects as if they owned them? And her life too! A nurse! Contemptible!' (p. 49).

The problem of self-realization in later life affects both carers and those for whom they feel responsible. In *At Paradise Gate* Ike the invalid suspects (correctly) that he is being talked about behind his back, and in *Family Money* Nina Bawden gives us access to the private family discussion among Fanny Pye's children after she has been hospitalized following an attack in the street and is (temporarily it turns out) shaken and confused. In anticipation of Fanny's decline they debate the effects of the injury on her health and her long-term mental state, and discuss how she will best be cared for in the future. When she discovers what has been going on, Fanny is angered at what she considers to be her children talking behind her back and making mistaken assumptions about her frailty; she feels 'outraged and fearful' (Bawden 1997: 52). Later, in bed, she compares her condition with that of childhood 'in which all adults were enemies in league with each other, talking over her head and sealing her fate without ever consulting her'. Old people, though she does not see herself as old, 'were helpless as children' (p. 52).

Fanny's descent into physical dependency and mental confusion is only temporary and the novel goes on to show how she makes a full recovery and resumes control of her life. The attack is a temporary setback and not the beginning of an unremitting decline, and is an interesting example of how physical injury shifts the balance of power between children and parents and produces anticipatory ageing. It also shows how the motives of people who believe they have a duty to care for the older members of the family may be mixed: the concern of Fanny's children over her future welfare is coloured by their appreciation of the market value of her London house and their anticipated inheritance

The shifting balances of power associated with dependency are also evident in Vita Sackville-West's *All Passion Spent*. Lady Slane, the central character, is widowed and a family discussion takes place early in the novel about her future care. In her children's eyes the death of their father has made Lady Slane dependent on them; she cannot possibly live alone. But these children, themselves middle aged, have neglected the fact that widowhood can for a short period transfer the power of the father as head of this aristocratic household to the widow, and it is during this transitional period that Lady Slane decides to determine her own future through the purchase of a house in Hampstead she has dreamed of all her life, and by setting up an independent life with only her maid for company. There are plenty of older women, she announces to the amazement of her children, who: 'live in retirement at Hampstead. Besides, I have considered the eyes of the world for so long that I think it is time I had a little holiday from them. If one is not to please oneself in old age, when is one to please oneself? There is so little time left!' (Sackville-West 1989: 66–7).

Fictional descriptions of shifts and changes in balances of power show how the identities of older people are shaped by the situations they find themselves in and their responses to these situations. The example of Lady Slane shows how what Cohen (1994: 99) has described as the determination in later life 'to be self-directing' requires the older person to make changes in the relationships which are central to his or her changing sense of selfhood. By removing herself from the family mansion, Lady Slane creates a new distance between her children and herself and makes the transition from the domestic role of perpetual family carer to one of independent selfhood on her own terms. Significantly, the self she wishes to express is related to a particular place: the house she first saw 30 years ago and all those years ago identified as '*her* house' (Sackville-West 1989: 87). Moving house symbolizes a radical break with social expectations concerning the proper way for aristocratic ladies to age in England during the 1920s. Lady Slane rejects the restrictions of the grandmother or 'grannie' role and chooses to grow older on her own terms. Before she dies her final act of rebellion is to give approval to her great-granddaughter's wish to become a musician.

Conversations

Research shows that conversations between younger and older people are frequently characterized by the use of terms of 'age categorization' (Coupland *et al*. 1991). In their linguistic analysis of intergenerational conversations, Coupland *et al*. begin with the assumption that the language we use in conversations is influenced by specific situations, and in turn influences individual perceptions. Age awareness is thus shaped through the words we use in conversation and our choice of words is influenced by the situation and the expectation different age groups have of each other.

When younger and older people meet there is an expectation that age will be a relevant conversational topic, and it can be introduced in a number of ways. In conversations, age identity is constructed through a number of age categorization processes, which include: the disclosure of chronological age; reference to age-related categories such as 'pensioner', 'geriatric', and 'old' through, for example, the use of phrases such as 'I have to pay for that myself and I'm a pensioner' (Coupland *et al*. 1991: 60); and reference to age identity in terms of health, physical decline and death. In addition, there are a number of 'temporal framing processes' in which a time perspective is introduced into the conversation. These include: references to experiences which have taken place in the past; places lived in and visited in the past; associating the self with the past; and drawing attention to change, when, for example, someone says 'in those days you had to work hard to make ends meet because you had no money' (Coupland *et al*. 1991: 65). In summary, therefore, these forms of age categorization can involve the 'disclosure of chronological age, generational/family role or other age-related role reference' and also the use of 'discursive framing, as when an older speaker talks about the past and thus identifies himself/herself temporally' (Ylanne-McEwen 1999: 419).

Because much of fiction describes sequences of face-to-face interaction, stories of ageing provide insight into the ways in which age consciousness is shaped during the course of a conversation. Conversations are one medium through which the self has the potential to develop through language in relation to others. An interesting example occurs in Stanley Middleton's *Beginning To End*, which opens with an accidental encounter between two characters we have already met, Anthony Clark, who is a young teacher in a private school, and Ernest Stapleton. As Clark is walking down a street one day he catches sight of a man who has dropped his shopping on the pavement and is leaning against the wall. Coming closer he can see that the man is 'elderly' and having trouble with his breathing; he offers to give him a hand with his carrier bags and accompanies him back to his house. Stapleton is clearly someone whose body has let him down. When his daughter Jennifer arrives she thanks Clark and tells him that her father has angina and is ' "tiptoeing around the margins of life" ' (Middleton 1991: 7). She asks Clark if he will visit her father again because he will benefit from the stimulus of conversation with a younger person, and the two men appear to have something in common:

> 'He'd be pleased. These days he seems very unsure of himself. You were swapping quotations, weren't you? He'd like that. His memory's going, but the bits and pieces of learning he picked up at school seem to stay with him. If you visit him again, throw a bit of Latin or Greek in; he'd like that.'
>
> (Middleton 1991: 7)

Stapleton, she says, has few friends and has difficulty in seeing his daughter as anything but a child. Clark agrees (he is also attracted to Jennifer) and as a result of this chance encounter the relationship between Clark and Stapleton develops so that almost at the end of the novel there are signs that Stapleton is making small changes in his attitude to life and is communicating more openly. Jennifer describes a recent meeting she has had with her father who has been to a funeral. He has made an effort to take care with his appearance and he speaks 'seriously' with her in a way he would not have done before because he was brought up in a world where men did not normally confide in their daughters. He is not grumbling as much as usual about noisy neighbours, and the idleness of the younger generation, and he raises the question of the meaning of life. It was not, Jennifer says, 'very enlightening, but at least he was trying to express himself to me. I feel a bit touched by it now' (Middleton 1991: 223).

Two days later, Stapleton is dead from a heart attack. There were no further developments in this small-scale change in the relationship between father and daughter, but the shift displayed in Stapleton's transition towards more open self-disclosure is an indication of the subtle ways attitudes to ageing may change over a period of time and are expressed in everyday conversation. One of the contributions of the novelist to our understanding of the ageing process is to create those nuanced sequences of social interaction which are so difficult to observe and record in conventional gerontological research.

In Middleton's *Necessary Ends*, Sam Martin, aged 81, and retired to a bungalow in a Norfolk seaside village, becomes friendly by chance with a couple in their thirties, Karen and Edward Craig, who are on holiday with their children. They first meet after Martin has by chance discovered the small young daughter who is lost, and he brings them back together. The ensuing development of this relationship enables the novelist to introduce intergenerational conversations around the subject of the experience of ageing. Shortly after their first meeting Martin invites the family to his home when he casually mentions in a discussion of gardening and fruit that 75 years have passed since his mother gave him sugar in a paper to dip his rhubarb in. This passing reference to his childhood prompts a further exchange about his age:

'You're exaggerating,' Mrs Craig said.
'Exaggerating what?' he asked.
'Your age.'
'I'm eighty-one.' . . .
'I should have guessed you were early sixties at most,' the mother said. 'What do you think, Ted?'
'No more than that,' he answered.
'That's flattering,' the old man answered. 'It feels otherwise.'
(Middleton 1999: 14)

Conversational exchanges between younger and older characters show how the problem of describing the experience of ageing arises out of the symbolic significance of the chronological distance that exists between younger and older people. The story of *Necessary Ends* is constructed to show Sam in relationships with characters of different ages including Alice Jeffreys, who is in her sixties, yet is still seeing herself as sufficiently removed from Sam's 81 years to ask the question ' "What's it like being old?" ' (p. 58). In his reply Sam describes a distinction between his experience of the body and his awareness of a self which is grounded in a particular period of history:

'I've got all my hair. And I'm not too wrinkled or fat. But I feel my age. Not in aches and pains. I'm fortunate there. . . . No, it's not physically but in my head. The world seems to have left me behind. . . . That's terrifying. All that time has gone, slipped away, disappeared. Things that happened more than seventy years ago are as vivid as yesterday's or last year's affairs. I've been left behind.'
(Middleton 1999: 58–9)

Conversations between individuals of different ages are a notable feature in a number of Stanley Middleton's novels. In *Brief Hours* the central character is Frank Stapleton, a successful accountant who has retired. He is married to Thelma and their son's marriage to Francesca is going through troubled times. In spite of the tensions between their married children, Frank and Thelma still maintain friendly relations with their son's in-laws and a significantly age identifying conversation occurs when they accompany Sarah, their daughter-in-law's mother on a visit to her own mother who is aged 87 and in private residential care. The old woman does not now recognize her daughter and her inability to communicate prompts the following exchange between Frank, Thelma and Sarah as they drive back home:

'Did her condition come on her suddenly?' Thelma, again.
'No. Well. She became forgetful in her late seventies. Vague. And by the time she was eighty-odd it wasn't safe to leave her on her own. She's become much worse since she came in here four years ago. She's eighty-seven now. It's a big age. Even these days.'
(Middleton 1997: 148)

When remembered in her fifties, Sarah's mother was 'energetic' (p. 148); 'She knew her mind then' (p. 149). ' "And to see her now." That sobered them quickly enough. "She doesn't even look the same. She was a broad, well-set up woman, strong. . . . Now she's quite different, like a skeleton. I wouldn't recognise her" ' (p. 149). Later, Thelma says ' "It's thirty-one, thirty-two years ago since Francesca [her daughter] started school. In thirty-two years I shall be older than my mother is now. I hope I don't live that long. Good God" ' (p. 149).

In positioning Frank between his son, daughter-in-law, grandchildren, and the old, confused lady in residential care, Middleton is clearly drawing on the traditional imagery of life as a series of relationships between generations who represent the 'ages' and 'stages' of life. And it is through the medium of conversation that these images of past, present and future are brought to life. Not only does Sarah's mother appear to have lost her mind, and therefore her independent self, her body is no longer recognizable. Her body and self in the present and the future can only be connected with her body and self in the past through an effort of the imagination.

Age-discrepant relationships

Age identity emerges out of perceived contrasts between members of different age groups and this can be fraught with particular tensions when the relationships are sexual, or at least one of the parties wishes this were so.

In *The Wench is Dead*, Colin Dexter's Inspector Morse is taken into the John Radcliffe Hospital in Oxford suffering from a perforated ulcer. On two occasions the unmarried, middle-aged and romantically-minded Morse comes to see himself as he imagines the young nurses see him. On admission to hospital his preliminary examination is carried out by a young nurse and he notices the difference in the quality of the interaction when she is engaged with a casualty of a rugby match who is covered in mud from the field and, more importantly, young:

> Morse could do little but envy the familiarity that was affected forthwith between the young lad and the equally young lass. Suddenly – and almost cruelly – Morse realised that she, that same young lass, had seen him – Morse! – for exactly what he was: a man who'd struggled through life to his early fifties, and who was about to face the slightly infra-dignitatem embarrassments of hernias and haemorrhoids, of urinary infections and yes! – of duodenal ulcers.
>
> (Dexter 1990: 5)

In quite a different novel, Julian Rathbone's *Blame Hitler*, Thomas Somers, almost 60 and on holiday without his family, picks up a young woman to whom he is sexually attracted. He takes her to a bullfight and as they discuss the rights and wrongs of bullfighting Somers expresses his view that although the bull is to be killed in the ring at least he has enjoyed a full life and is dying in his prime. He is spared the physical indignities of the decline that Somers anticipates as his lot in later life. Wouldn't you rather die, he asks, 'in the full glory of your womanhood . . . at the height of all your abilities' than live on to 'old age, cancer, with Alzheimer's as a side order after twenty years of merciless decline?' (Rathbone 1998: 194). Somers' depressing version of ageing as a 'decline narrative' is prompted by the memory of his mother's undignified disintegration. His personal vision of ageing is shaped out of the contrast between the youthful attraction of his companion, the memory of his mother, and his own sense of consciousness of middle age. Later he is described through the eyes of a young German hiker as a 'plump, almost elderly, Englishman' (p. 279).

The imaginative ability to see ourselves through the eyes of others may make ageing problematic for the older person in an age-discrepant relationship and is often unflattering. It is an example of the perils of 'unequal lovers', images of whom have been around for centuries (Stewart 1977). Some characters anticipate the stigma of ageing when they find themselves sexually attracted to younger people. At one point Somers compares himself unfavourably with a younger man, Pierre:

> At least fifteen years older than Pierre, and a degenerate, fat, old, balding wreck; why should she think such a thing? Probably she was remembering how he had gone to the downstairs loo that first dawn, mother-naked, half-drunk, pot-bellied with the smallest prick she'd ever seen. That's why she was grinning.
>
> (Rathbone 1998: 178)

In love affairs between younger and older partners the negotiation of the meaning of ageing and its implications for the relationship is in fiction usually even more emotionally intense and consequential, as Joanna Trollope, for example, shows in *The Men and the Girls*. The central interest in this novel is the intimate relationships between two younger women and their partners, who are much older men. In this context the novelist is freer than the research gerontologist to imagine the subjective dimensions of various permutations in relationships between younger and older people, and also to display the ways in which perceptions of ageing may be used as an expression of change in the attitudes of one of the partners. In the following incident, James Mallow, a retired teacher, is telling his young partner Kate Bain how he has knocked an older woman off her bicycle because he had forgotten his spectacles when he took the car out. The woman is not badly hurt but the incident has upset him and he expects Kate to comfort him:

> But she didn't. She said nothing and she didn't move. He looked across at her, surprised. She was regarding him with a look that was wholly unfamiliar, a cold contemptuous look.
> He opened his mouth to speak but before he could utter, Kate said in a voice that matched her expression, 'You stupid old man.' Then there was another silence, in which they regarded each other with horror.
>
> (Trollope 1993: 18)

This incident in the early pages of the novel marks the beginning of their awareness that a relationship which has lasted apparently comfortably for eight years is beginning to change and is in the early stages of decline. This awareness is expressed at first in Kate's ageist language which is the outward and almost involuntary expression of a growing awareness of a deeper incompatibility. In this instance age discrepancy, hitherto unproblematic and even a source of positive emotions, takes a negative turn and becomes an increasing source of tension once it has been so suddenly and so crudely articulated. As the novel unfolds so the age difference becomes an increasingly important issue between James and Kate. Shortly after her disconcerting rebuke, Kate takes a bath where she broods over its implications. For she sees James in all other respects as a kind and thoughtful partner whose age had been if anything a 'turn-on' when they first met:

> . . . now she had called him a stupid old man, she realized with a shock that she meant it. It *was* the behaviour of a stupid, myopic, absent-minded old man to drive about in the dark and rain without glasses and knock people off bicycles. Oh God, thought Kate, suddenly afraid of where her mind was going, what am I doing?
>
> (Trollope 1993: 19)

Awareness of the signs of ageing in others or, as in the case of Kate, interpretations of signs of ageing in James' minor motor accident, exercises a reflexive influence over conceptions of the self. In labelling James as a 'stupid old man' Kate has produced a reassessment of herself. She later apologizes to James and he accepts her apology with the comment that her reaction is probably correct – but their relationship is never the same again.

In *The Actresses* by Barbara Ewing, Molly is suddenly informed by her younger lover Banjo that he has to leave her because he wants children and she is too old (Ewing 1997: 275–6). A love affair between a younger man and an older woman where the differences in ages appeared to be entirely acceptable and even a cause for self-congratulation on Molly's part is suddenly undermined and brought to an end by the passing of time and the changing expectations of the younger partner. Following this experience, Molly's self-conception can never be quite the same again.

In quite a different example from non-fiction, a father and daughter relationship, Linda Grant (1998) recalls with honesty and regret the changes she experienced in her attitude towards her father as she grew into a teenager and he grew older. She recounts the combination of feelings of embarrassment and disgust his appearance and illness aroused in her when he was in his sixties, and how the two gradually grew apart. The man whose style and physical appearance signalled desirable qualities of fatherhood to a 7-year-old girl was transformed in her teenage eyes into a pathetic and self-indulgent old man:

> Later, in the long years of his illness, I could not stay in the room at mealtimes to see him fall asleep over the dinner table, his mouth hanging open with food still in it. He more than embarrassed me, he disgusted me. I hated the years of his decline, his petty addictions to food and alcohol and gambling. . . . When I was seven I was in love with him, demanding that he take me to the theatre and treat me as his date, buy me a box of chocolates as once he had sent me little posies of anemones, tucked into my mother's larger bouquets. But when I grew up I wanted a thin, young, long-haired boyfriend. Not a fat, bald, sixty-year-old.
>
> (Grant 1998: 72–3)

In these episodes a younger person's perception of the ageing of a close relation or partner produces embarrassment and is an impediment to smooth and harmonious social interaction. Embarrassing incidents cause strains in relationships which, as in the fictitious example of Kate and James may lead to a deeper rift, or as in Linda Grant's biographical account, are remembered with regret. When associated with ageing, embarrassing incidents and changes in appearance are often evaluated morally: James is not simply accused by Kate of being an 'old man' but a '*stupid* old man', words that in combination add a measure of blame to an assessment of mental competence and chronological age.

What this variety of examples shows is that age identity emerges out of interaction between younger and older people, although the interpretation of age differences will vary according to the nature of the relationship, its history, situation, place and the passage of time. The main character in Penelope Lively's *City of the Mind* is Mathew Halland, an architect working in London. Mathew is comparatively young but his awareness of ageing is fostered by the appearance of his widowed mother who he sees as 'withered – there is less of her each year, he feels' (Lively 1992: 50) and by his feeling that her use of the popular expression ' "We're none of us getting any younger" ' now includes 'him in the sweep' (p. 98). He feels himself to be in some way in a transitional state signified by his mother's references to his pension arrangements and her ambiguously 'treating him as a peer' while still 'according him the licence due to youth' (p. 99).

The role of interaction in shaping consciousness of ageing in the self and others is evident in the choice of words used in conversations, in bodily gestures and facial expressions. One of the ways that ageing is constructed in social interaction is through talk (Coupland *et al.* 1991; Ylanne-McEwen 1999). As we have seen from the bruising incident when Kate called James 'a stupid old man' (*The Men and the Girls*), and in the way in which Mathew Halland's mother now includes him in the expression 'We're none of us getting any younger' (*The City of The Mind*), age identity is *shaped* through conversations. As Virpi Ylanne-McEwen shows in her analysis of interaction between older customers and assistants in a travel agency: 'the experience of ageing and later life is lived through face-to-face interaction' (1999: 437).

Secrets

One of the considerable advantages of fiction, as we have seen, is that it allows the reader access to the subjective perceptions of all the parties in a particular sequence of social interaction. It illuminates the complex interaction between self and other which is central to the symbolic interactionist perspective on ageing. However, because, as Goffman (1968, 1969) has shown, interaction is about the amount of information we reveal to others about ourselves, there is the problem of secrets. All human interaction raises the problem of information management and ageing may bring particular problems in this respect. Linda Grant (1998) describes how the problem with Alzheimer's disease is not only the physical loss of friends and family, who may momentarily appear, but also the problem of whether or not we knew the person in the past. Here, family secrets come into play. How do we 'know' another person?

How much does one party to interaction reveal to another? Secrets, as Vaughan (1988) has shown, are a significant part of the self. At the end of Henry Sutton's *Gorleston*, Percy has discovered a distressing secret about his wife's past life which everyone else in his circle seemed to share. The revelation of his wife's secret love for another man turns his world upside down. He now sees his memories of events in the past in a completely different light and he is left with the bitter realization that his marriage had been a failure and a sham. Not only is the past as remembered now utterly changed, but the present and the future and the stability of Percy's sense of selfhood is undermined. He comes to see that his memory of his wife was based upon an illusion; how could he have really known her, for she secretly cherished love for another man? The realization that his knowledge of his wife's emotional life was flawed reflects back on Percy's confidence in his own knowledge of himself: he 'no longer felt he knew himself. He felt a great gap open up inside him. A great void. The void was a grey, a greeny-grey, the colour of the sea. He felt he was being enveloped by it' (Sutton 1995: 244).

In *The Road to Lichfield*, Penelope Lively explores the issue of family secrets in her story about Anne Linton whose father, James, aged 80, has been admitted into hospital in a serious condition. Anne, who is married with a family and lives in the South of England is now linked with her father by the road to Lichfield which she has to travel to visit him. James has been a widower for ten years, and is in a confused state, suffering from Parkinson's disease, a weak heart and incontinence. Now that her father is no longer in control of his situation and is not expected to live, Anne has also to spend time in his house going through his affairs. As she checks through what was once his private home and papers, she discovers a mysterious regular payment to a Mrs Barron in Gloucester.

Her discovery of the mysterious payment takes us to the heart of the distance that can separate social from subjective selves even in the close intimacy of family life. Anne begins to reinterpret the past, discovering that her father had a mistress and that her brother was party to the secret. Eventually, she meets Mrs Barron who turns out to be the middle-aged daughter of her father's mistress, Betty Mansell. Shirley Barron's mother has been dead for nine years and Anne, who wishes to know more about her father and his other life, asks her what they used to talk about. This new knowledge of her father's secret life forces Anne to reflect on the quality of the intimate relationships between her father, who is now fading away, and the two dead women to whom he apparently expressed different selves. As the novel unfolds, Anne becomes more aware of the symbolic power of the dead to influence the living:

> They are all, Anne thought, either dead or beyond remembering what happened. Mother. Mrs Mansell. Father. But because of them we sit here, two people otherwise unconnected, talking about something that is only our affair at one remove, and yet, somehow matters very much to both of us.
>
> (Lively 1983: 148)

Anne's experience, of course, is an emotional one and the emotions surrounding ageing are a significant ingredient in stories of ageing. Fiction is particularly adept at describing and expressing the emotions associated with growing older. Part of the feeling that is aroused is in the contrast between what individuals were formerly and what they have now become.

For the novelist the narrative potential of secrets is such that the discovery of hidden complexities in the character of a person who has the stereotypical appearance of old age is not necessarily a pleasant one. The view of the individual as 'a basket of selves which come to the surface at different social moments' (Cohen 1994: 11) brings the possibility of the individual's awareness of a number of selves hidden from the view of the present audience. One of the attractions of using older characters in fiction is the possibility that they may harbour guilty secrets.

A good example is Lesley Glaister's *The Private Parts of Women* which is a disturbing story of multiple selves in old age. Inis, a young doctor's wife, runs away from her husband and children to a 'dreary little house in a dreary post-industrial city' (Glaister 1996: 1), where her next door neighbour is Trixie Bell, 84 years old and on the face of things a rather ordinary older woman. She has a face which Inis would like to photograph because it is 'beautifully old and she has a sort of dignity' (p. 18). At first the only discordant note is the vigorous sound of her voice singing hymns penetrating through the adjoining wall:

> a loud, strong, woman's voice and the thump of a beat, maybe her foot on the floor. It could only have been Trixie, though I would not have thought such a voice would come from her, she looks so done in, sort of defeated. 'Onward Christian Soldiers' she sang, and 'He Who Would Valiant Be'
>
> (Glaister 1996: 19)

As the story unfolds, Inis penetrates deeper into the privacy of Trixie's home and discovers to her cost the multiple selves and threatening selves concealed behind the façade of a stereotypically nonedescript old age.

Loneliness and exclusion

Loneliness is closely associated with social exclusion and isolation and is a powerfully emotive term because it arises, as Linda A. Wood (1988) has shown, from the experience of 'the absence of human connections' (p. 184). But the absence of human connections is more than the experience of living in physical or geographical isolation from other people – the stereotype of the older widow living, for example, in the depths of the countryside. Wood develops the definition of loneliness to refer explicitly to what she calls 'the individual experience of *failed* intersubjectivity' (p. 188), by which she means a failure in 'mutual understanding' – a lack of a sense that there is someone else who shares one's experience. In this definition, individuals are not necessarily physically isolated from other people, but an individual person feels lonely when the inner sense of selfhood is experienced as disconnected or excluded from links with other people with whom she or he closely identifies or would like to identify.

The lonely individual is therefore 'aware of not sharing the same taken-for-granted meanings' as others (Wood 1988: 188). The lonely individual experiences a sense of separation from other people and 'an absence of shared understanding' (p. 189). In this sense, one can be in the company of others and still feel the emotion of loneliness: 'One of the respondents in my research with the rural elderly [Wood 1981] reported that the loneliest time in her life was when she was forced by circumstances to have sustained interaction with a sister-in-law with whom she shared very few assumptions about the world' (1988: 189). In Paul Bailey's *At The Jerusalem*, Mrs Gadny has been found a place by her stepson and his wife in The Jerusalem, a former workhouse turned into 'a home for the elderly and dying' (Bailey 1987: 14). In the story readers are invited to identify with Mrs Gadny from whose perspective The Jerusalem is seen as an alien environment into which she has been placed by her unsympathetic stepson and his wife. But we are also given a glimpse of how Mrs Gadny appears to Thelma, her stepson's wife, when she is living at her home. Thelma and Mrs Gadny's stepson regard her as depressed and depressing, incontinent, confused and a disturbing influence on the children. She is therefore sent to The Jerusalem 'for her own good'. But in Mrs Gadny's experience, ageing is bringing isolation and exclusion from her social role and the people who gave her a sense of self-worth. She feels she has nothing in common with the other women in care. For her, The Jerusalem, is 'hell on earth' because there is no escape from the other inmates. They are constantly in each other's company; they sleep together in dormitories and:

> You turned a corner and the creature's yellow face above the tippet was coming for you. If you went to the toilet very soon someone would suspect you of doing something and either bang on or open the door. In the lounge – that hateful word – they sat about or slept with their mouths open. And, if they had eaten too much, they made noises and sometimes smells.
>
> (Bailey 1987: 80)

But at least at mealtimes, Mrs Gadny thinks, it is possible to turn your eyes away and focus your gaze on your plate.

Mrs Gadny tries to find some relief from her sense of isolation by confiding her experiences in letters to her friend Mrs Barber. But Mrs Barber never replies; she has, we discover, been dead for two years and it is her daughter who receives and opens the letters, and dismisses their contents. Mrs Gadny's personal anguish also leads her to look inside herself for symbolic sources of support for her self-image. She retreats into her memories for solace and for that reason is perceived by the staff to be displaying an uncooperative attitude. The gradual process of exclusion from the world of the compliant and therefore contented inmate ends with her being defined as mad and ironically isolated from the others in a private room. At The Jerusalem only the antisocial are given privacy.

Dorothy Jerrome has defined intimate relationships as 'characterised by emotional intensity, self-disclosure and a high degree of personal involvement' (1993: 226). Such relationships need not necessarily be harmonious and the fiction on relationships in 'homes' for old people tends to find narrative power in stories of rivalry and conflict. Rivalry and conflict may include the value placed on others who see that a resident has frequent visitors and has not been abandoned by family and friends. Living in residential accommodation means sustaining a presentation of a social self before an audience. When meals are taken in public and much of social life takes place in a public setting, then a performance must be sustained. Visitors are of course a reminder that life was not always like this and that the resident who is now older should not be dismissed as being of no consequence; there is the important issue of saving face at stake.

In Elizabeth Taylor's *Mrs Palfrey at The Claremont*, the hotel is structured in terms of a series of social gradations: Mrs Palfrey feels socially inferior to Lady Swayne, who dines at the Savoy, but socially superior to Mrs Burton, who is 'not the sort of woman . . . with whom she would ordinarily have been in company' (Taylor 1996: 15). Mrs Palfrey's grandson and heir Desmond, whom she has deliberately mentioned in conversation and for whom she is publicly knitting to show the others she is not alone in the world, works in the British Museum. But her social status is threatened because he repeatedly fails to visit her. 'Relations', says Mrs Post, 'make all the difference. . . . Although one would never make a home with them' (p. 10). At first Mrs Palfrey makes excuses for her grandson:

> Saving face had been an important part of life in the Far East, and Mrs Palfrey tried to save hers now. Trouble usually comes from doing so, and it came to her, for it involved her in telling lies, and in being obliged to remember the lies when she had told them. She had to invent illnesses for Desmond, and trips abroad connected with his work. . . . She found this a great strain, and along with it went her secret grief that she had no one of her own in London after all, and that the studious, rather prim young man she had always been proud of seemed utterly unconcerned about her.
>
> (Taylor 1996: 18)

Eventually, Mrs Palfrey is drawn into the pretence that a young man she has encountered by chance after she turned her ankle and fell in the street is her grandson. This is Ludo, a struggling writer, who helped her to her feet and took her into his dingy flat to restore her. As a reward she invites him to dinner at the more affluent Claremont. When she announces to the waiter, 'well within Mrs Arbuthnot's hearing' (p. 32), that she is expecting a guest to dinner, Mrs Arbuthnot jumps to the conclusion that it is her grandson 'and, for some reason she searched for later, Mrs Palfrey let her go without a word' (p. 32). Having embarked on the deception, Mrs Palfrey carries it through, asking Ludo if he minds whether she calls him Desmond. Ludo, who is poor, goes along with this because he is getting free meals in a good hotel. But another pay-off for Ludo is the opportunity the dinners provide for the cold-blooded observation of Mrs Palfrey's behaviour. He is writing a novel about 'elderly women' and Mrs Palfrey unwittingly has become a resource (p. 48).

The death of others

Our discussion so far has considered fictional representations of the interaction between the self and others in terms of relationships with living people.

While the experience of loneliness or subjective exclusion can occur at any time of life, one of the problems of ageing is that it is often accompanied by physical separation, due to death, from those with whom we identify most closely. In the final pages of Stanley Middleton's *Necessary Ends* Sam Martin calls into his village pub for a drink and is told of the unexpected death of Jack Brentnall, a fellow retiree with whom he had struck up an acquaintance. Although the two had not been close friends Sam is upset by this news – a 'tear trickled down his face from his left eye', he experiences a constriction in his throat and his arms hang 'leaden.' (Middleton 1999: 216). The two men had liked each other, had shared a sense of common background and a similar view of the outside world. The disappearance of others with whom one shares this kind of bond, Sam reflects, comes as a sharp, and in his case unwelcome, reminder of the 'transience of the world' (p. 216).

As linguistic research shows, conversations between generations are often routinely drawn to the ageing body and its associations with illness and death (Coupland *et al.* 1991). In another novel by Stanley Middleton, *Live and Learn*, a conversation takes place between Alfred Perkins, aged around 50, and Jonathan Winter, aged 28. Perkins, a middle-aged man positioned between his father and his son, tells Winter that his father is dying of cancer:

> 'He's at home. That's a good thing. He gets MacMillan nurses and all the rest; they're very good. He's in no serious pain, only discomfort, utter weakness. He can't do anything for himself. He doesn't eat, but just lies or sits there, not a bit of flesh on him, and he was a man of my size.'
>
> Perkins slapped his paunch.
>
> 'How old is he?'
>
> 'Seventy-two.' Perkins moved his mouth round. 'It's past three score years and ten, but it's not old these days. And I see him there. He's no voice left. He understands what people say, and that it only needs a bit of chest infection and he's done, gone.'
>
> 'Is he clinging on to life?'
>
> 'No. I don't think he is. He'd be glad to go, I reckon. He's doing no good to himself, to my mother, to anybody. He has no religious beliefs. He's stuck there, weak as water, waiting. He can barely get his tablets down him. He isn't angry he's too weak. But he sees me there, and he looks at me. I hold his hand, but he's ashamed of that.'
>
> (Middleton 1996: 23)

Perkins' father, as described in the above passage is now obsolete, his present self has no voice and he is embarrassed by any other expressions of emotion. Contact between the two men has apparently been almost severed by the demands of the declining body and the self seems to have disappeared as the body becomes a dominating force. The description by Perkins of his father's 'dys-appearing body' is also a reminder to younger observers of the precarious nature of physical health – that the absent body should not be taken for granted. Perkins slaps his own paunch to draw attention to his father's previously embodied self: 'he was a man of my size'. But we learn that Perkins himself is to die soon after his father; prematurely, of a heart attack. And Winter later wonders whether Perkins, during what was to be their last conversation, was unconsciously aware that 'the best' of his life, too, was nearly over and that in the future he 'must live through other people' (p. 81).

Renewed contact with figures from the past may also stimulate age consciousness and awareness of age identity. In *Toward the Sea*, Stanley Middleton provides his central character, Henry Shelton aged 59, with an unexpected encounter with Marion Ball, a former lover. It is over 40 years since they last met when she, five years older, initiated him into sex. Marion's daughter, Helena, has contacted Henry out of the blue and arranged a meeting with her mother who has been very ill: she has, says Helena, spoken of him many times and Henry now waits at Helena's house to see Marion again:

> He recalled Marion, the violent young woman with the wet mouth, the searching hands, and wondered what he would find now. Again the door opened, slowly this time, and Marion Ball eased her way in, guided from the crook of her arm by Helena. She walked upright and firmly, unlike a sick person, but stood at first inside the room, partially excluding her daughter.
> 'Here's Mr Shelton,' Helena called in a bright, social voice.
> 'Henry.' Marion extended her hand. He stepped forward to grasp it. 'It's a long time. But I would have recognised you.'
> He would not have recognised her, would have passed her in the street. The face seemed thin, lined, haggard with recent illness. Her hands were ugly, knotted, thickly spotted. She had dressed fashionably, as though she could afford the time and money, and in youthful colours, which suited her for she had not grown fat or shapeless.
>
> (Middleton 1995: 13)

This meeting between Henry and Marion stimulates Henry's awareness of ageing by provoking his memory and fusing together past, present and future in one single encounter. In his mind Henry compares his memories of Marion's embodied self in the distant past with her present appearance. As a woman who 'flaunted her sex' she had broken the 'provincial conventions of love' and 'lifted him into an ecstasy beyond price'. But 'now she was a smartly dressed skeleton with barely a word to offer him' (p. 19).

When a person dies, memories are left behind and interaction with the living may continue into the future. The self may become symbolically detached from the body and the symbolic characteristics of identity may linger long after the body has died. There is research evidence that although they may be reluctant to discuss their experiences openly, a number of widows have a strong sense of the continuing presence of their dead husbands:

> . . . we are disturbed by the ongoing social presence of individuals who are dead. Indeed, those whose daily lives continue to be lived out in what they regard as intimate proximity to deceased partners or children, have, until recently, been diagnosed as suffering from 'pathological grief'.
>
> (Hallam *et al.* 1999: 11)

In addition, therefore, to the images of persons no longer physically present preserved in photographs, letters and other memorabilia, the disembodied interactions of the dead with the living include ghostly hauntings, spiritualist seances and other paranormal phenomena. In short, the others with whom individual selves identify do not have to be physically present to provide interactive support and to keep the 'failed intersubjectivity' of loneliness at bay. The inner sense of selfhood is symbolically integrated with others whose presence may be invisible to other observers. The self that Mead described as a conversation is thus kept alive in the imagination.

Places can be haunted by the memory of the dead, persisting in the structure and design of the home and in the biographical objects it contains. Because the self, the 'I' and the 'me', consists of patterns of social interaction which are part of the structure of our mental lives, the influence of others who have died can continue subjectively in the form of remembered conversations, or voices in the head.

A particularly good example occurs in Penelope Lively's *Passing On* which begins with the funeral of Dorothy Glover, a tyrannical woman, who has died at the age of 80. Her daughter Helen and son Edward are now middle-aged and have lived with her for 30 years. But her death does not bring an immediate end to her dominant role in their lives. Their problem is that they cannot shake off the memory of the way she has regulated their entire existence. Reminders of Dorothy's influence linger on in the decaying structure of the house (aptly named 'Greystones'), its decorations, furnishings, kitchen utensils and her accumulated clothing. In symbolic terms Helen and Edward are haunted both in their physical situation and within their own heads by Dorothy's ghost. Throughout the novel Dorothy is an imagined presence who persists symbolically in the imprint she has left on the furnishings, the décor of the house, in the material evidence of her past authoritarian actions, but ultimately even more forcefully in the impression she has left in the minds of Helen and Edward:

> From time to time she [Helen] saw Greystones as others must see it. . . .
> The cracks in the flagged floor. The green mould creeping up the wall by
> the back door that one just ignored because if you redecorated it simply
> crept up again within a month or two. The rusting cake tins. The crockery. That sink.
>
> (Lively 1989: 32)

Later, Helen takes her friend Giles Carnaby into the kitchen and in her mind's eye contrasts his warm and modernized kitchen with the sight before her of dripping taps, and decaying dishcloths: 'Like Dorothy, Helen and Edward used swabs of mouldering grey stockingette; they festered by the sink and were known as dead rabbits' (p. 132). ' "It has" ', she says to Carnaby, ' "a sort of museum appeal. One almost expects a mangle" ' (p. 132).

In Helen's mind, Dorothy is the 'other': herself as she imagines her mother sees her, and on whom she passes judgement – on her thoughts, hopes, and actions. And much of this disapproval relates to her age and negative age identity. Out shopping, Helen looks at a display of sweaters and hears the voice of her mother say ' "You can't wear that sort of thing. . . . It's too young for you. You're fifty-two. And too short and too fat" ' (p. 20). When she contemplates a romantic involvement with the suave solicitor Giles Carnaby

Helen's mother's voice assumes a tone of ridicule, cautioning her against the futility of her desires. After lunch with Carnaby Helen drives home accompanied in her imagination by Dorothy 'sitting squatly in the passenger seat' telling her 'she was fifty-two years old, no beauty and never had been and would do better to pull herself together and think about something else' (p. 53). And going through the cloakroom full of fusty clothing Helen finds in the pocket of one of her mother's old discarded jackets a letter sent by a boyfriend years ago. This has obviously been intercepted to put a stop to what Dorothy considered to be an undesirable relationship. Helen is shaken with emotion by this memory and her new-found knowledge of her mother's role in what at the time was for her a puzzling breakdown in the romance: 'At this precise moment, thought Helen, I hate my mother. It was a refreshing feeling – invigorating even. And worth indulging: it stifled other feelings' (p. 110).

Towards the end of the novel, Helen reveals her love to Giles Carnaby knowing – her mother's voice in her head tells her it is so – that he will not wish to become involved because he is basically a flirt who is committed only to himself. This proves to be the case and although he doesn't want to stop seeing Helen she decides to end the relationship and they part. Although Helen is upset she gradually adjusts to the parting, seeing it ultimately as a kind of victory leaving her free to move on. This small triumph is part of the process through which, as a middle-aged woman, she liberates herself from the dominating memory of her mother whose imagined presence begins to fade and whose imagined voice is stilled. At the end of the novel, small but significant changes are taking place in Helen and Edward's lives. On the surface things apparently remain the same but Helen has started to think of making changes to the house and Edward will plant new trees in the ground behind the house: 'Everything was the same again, and yet was not' (p. 210). The ageing of both Helen and Edward is quietly positive: a gradual movement, viewed from their subjective perspective, towards some degree of personal autonomy and self-realization.

4

Objects, places and spaces

'Biographical objects'

In the previous chapter we looked at fictional representations of the ways in which the experience of ageing is expressed and given meaning during social interaction with others. In the last section of the chapter we also saw how significant others need not necessarily be living human beings. The repertoire of 'others' may be symbolically extended to include individuals who are no longer physically present, yet continue to play a significant role in supporting conceptions of the self and form a type of insulation against the 'failed intersubjectivity' of the loneliness often associated with later life. Because the self is a symbolic construct it can find support through an imaginative identification with people who are no longer physically alive. We also saw that interaction is situated, that it unfolds in particular places (for example, a retirement home, a community in a seaside town) and is structured by these material environments. In this chapter we look at the extension of the dependence of the individual self on others from living human beings to material objects and the places and spaces where individuals live and with which they are identified.

In their sociological analysis of the history of the English middle-class family Davidoff and Hall (1987) reproduce an amateur painting of the early nineteenth-century interior of an Essex farmhouse, showing an old woman situated at her typical place by the fireside. She inclines slightly towards the fireplace, knitting resting on her knees, and there is a contemplative look on her face. In keeping with the age-related costume of the period she is dressed from head to toe in black, her face encircled by a bonnet and fringed by a white cap beneath. She is, we are informed, a farmer's widow 'surrounded by paraphernalia of the middle class home: barometer, paintings, patterned wallpaper, brass fender and carpets' (p. 358). Another way of putting this is to say that the farmer's widow derives her identity in this picture from an appropriate arrangement of what have been described as 'biographical objects'. Biographical objects such as domestic possessions are 'entangled in the events of a person's life and used as a vehicle for a sense of selfhood' (Hoskins 1998: 2). When Victor Meldrew, the central character in David Renwick's *One Foot in The Grave*, returns from a holiday abroad to find his house burned down, all that remains identifiable in the rubble are the charred remnants of his childhood teddy bear. Although badly burnt, the face of the bear is still recognizable and because of the special place it occupies in Victor's memory of the past it has immeasurable value: 'Its true significance lay in something far more profound . . . deeply rooted in our own transience; in the acknowledgement of Time and times now lost for ever' (Renwick 1992: 81). The ruined bear is for Victor a cherished biographical object.

In 1995 the *Daily Mail* carried the story of a woman aged 85 who asked for her teddy bear to be cremated with her after her death. She had spent her last eight years in a nursing home in Bristol where she received no visitors. Her only companion was a large teddy bear she called 'Teddy Edward'. According to the report in the *Daily Mail* (1995) the teddy bear had been given to her as a child and two photographs of her with the bear were reproduced which showed her at the age of 3 and over 80 years later under the caption 'Inseparable'. Apparently little was known about her, she had few possessions and received no visitors: 'Her bear', said the owner of the nursing home, 'was her partner in life and in death' (*Daily Mail* 1995: 25).

At one level this story can be read as another poignant and stereotypical newspaper account of the loneliness and pathos of old age. But on another level it can be read alongside the Victor Meldrew story as evidence of the ability of human beings to form relationships with inanimate objects – in this case a toy – which sustain their subjective identity. We shall, of course, never know what 'Teddy Edward' meant to its owner but the photographs suggest that it ('he') provided 'his' owner, as in the fictional figure of Victor Meldrew, links to her past and some symbolic support for her sense of personal continuity over a long period of time and changing circumstances.

The overtones of pathos in this story are closely linked to the stereotypical view of old age as lonely. Human interest is also generated by the mixture of pathetic and infantilizing associations with childhood in terms of symbolic interaction with a furry toy. The *Daily Mail* story is truly sentimental, but it also reminds us of the important and often neglected fact that ageing is a complex emotional experience both for those who are growing older and for those who are looking on. Novelists are in a good position to draw on and develop the emotional content of social interaction in ways not always accessible to gerontological researchers.

Our capacity to give meaning to inanimate objects and to be moved emotionally by them connects us symbolically with the world of objects and places and extends the self beyond the boundaries of the material body. In Louise Doughty's *Honey-Dew* Alison, a young reporter on a local newspaper, visits Doug, her editor, in his bungalow. Doug, who is a widower, is in his fifties and has had a heart attack. When Alison sees inside his home for the first time she regards the sitting room as a 'backdrop' which provides material clues to Doug's status and his age identity:

His sitting room reeked of bachelorhood; the sad, middle-aged sort. On top of the television, there was a photograph of him and his late wife, an anniversary or some similar event. The silver frame was tarnished. Behind every eccentric, there is this backdrop, I thought; the woolly curtains that have never been washed, the gas fire. Scratch any *bon viveur* and you come up with a man who hasn't weighed himself for years because the idea of standing his loose white flesh on a pair of scales makes him want to burst into tears.

(Doughty 1999: 162)

Within places where people live we expect to find clues to their personal identity or what Gubrium (1995: 8) has described as: 'meaningfully available material objects'. In Mary Wesley's *Jumping the Queue*, Matilda Poliport, a widow, encounters Hugh, a much younger man who is on the run from the police. She tells Hugh that she and her husband Tom had agreed that when they grew older they would kill themselves to avoid the decrepitude of extreme old age and she intends, as she puts it, to 'tidy herself away':

'We decided we would leave no mess behind, nothing for the children to quarrel over. We would leave no messages, we would not let them know us once we were dead. Our children were not interested in how we had lived or felt, so our letters – when we were in love we wrote many letters, people did – we would destroy them. If they are ever interested it will be too late, we said.'

(Wesley 1991: 70)

However, Tom died unexpectedly, so Matilda is going to keep her side of the bargain. Hugh finds it hard to believe that Matilda is really closing down her life – has 'really swept herself away' (p. 87), and when she leaves him alone one day he searches the cottage for signs of her identity. There must, he thinks, 'be clues to her character that she was unconscious of leaving. He remembered exploring his home as a child, his discoveries among his parents' possessions' (p. 87).

Disposing of one's possessions can be seen as a voluntary form of 'social death', a process of separation from the world of the living prior to biological death. In other words it is the final social stage of disempowerment that Matilda Poliport and her husband were so anxious to avoid. In Nicci French's *The Memory Game*, an older and much loved character, Martha, prepares for her death from cancer by systematically tidying up all her papers and ordering her personal possessions:

On the morning of the funeral we looked through her drawers and wardrobes. Every item of clothing had been cleaned, folded and stowed. Some were in cardboard boxes with destinations marked in clear, assertive handwriting. Her workroom seemed empty but that was because it had been given a terminal organisation. . . . This was Martha's last great gesture. There was not a corner of the house where we could catch her ghost unawares in dishabille. Before she had departed she had left everything signed, sealed and as she wanted it.

(French 1998: 283)

There are close parallels here with the clergyman's widow, aged 92, inter-viewed by Ronald Blythe for his non-fiction portrayal of later life, *The View in Winter* (1981). She expresses a strong intention not to be a nuisance to those left behind when she has died. She doesn't want any more presents; is 'trying to get rid of things' and constantly tidying up. A stroke would mean she would lose control of her ability to organize her 'self' (1981: 317).

In David Cook's *Missing Persons*, Hetty Wainthrop, at the age of 70, sets up a private detective agency looking for missing persons. Hetty's friend Edith has a shoe-box of sepia photographs. This shoe-box is an interlinking theme throughout the story as Edith continually does a kind of reminiscence work, reviewing her past:

> Every memory she had of her early life contained within it her convic-tion then that she would never grow old. To be fifty had been unthink-able, and she would certainly never be so inconsiderate as still to be using up air, space and food at sixty, and seventy, but she had not grown old; only her body had done that. Her body had always betrayed her.
>
> (Cook 1988: 8)

Edith's younger self is preserved in her collection of old photographs which, at the end of the novel, she leaves to Hetty, her lifelong friend.

Personal possessions keep alive the sense of continuous selfhood through their symbolic association with events and people – what we sometimes describe as their 'sentimental value'. In this next example it is not a particu-lar object which is associated with the history of the self but the effort to remember where she has put it that stimulates Alice Matlock, an older char-acter in Peter Robinson's *Gallows View*, to reflect on her memories. She is trying to remember where she has put a sugar bowl, a present on her recent 87th birthday:

> Alice was having trouble remembering little things like that these days. They said it happened when you got older. But why, then, should the past seem so vivid? Why, particularly, should that day in 1916, when Arnold marched off so proudly to the trenches, seem so much clearer than yesterday. 'What happened yesterday?' Alice asked herself, as a test, and she did remember little details like visiting the shop, polishing her silverware and listening to a play on the radio. But had she really done those things yesterday, the day before, or even last week? The memories were there, but the string of time that linked them like a pearl necklace was broken. All those years ago – that beautiful summer when the meadows were full of buttercups (none of those nasty new bungalows then), the hedgerows bright with cow-parsley . . . and her garden full of roses, chrysanthemums, clematis and lupins – Arnold stood there, ready to go, his buttons reflecting the sunlight in dancing sparks on the white-washed walls. He leaned against the doorway, that very same doorway, with his kitbag and that lopsided grin on his face – such a young face, one that had never seen a razor – and off he marched, erect, graceful, to the station.
>
> (Robinson 1988: 2)

Objects, say Csikszentmihalyi and Rochberg-Halton (1981: 100), provide us with material evidence of 'how the self develops and is maintained across the life span', and in their research report on the meaning of 'things' they describe the home as a 'symbolic environment'. Their central point, drawing on interviews with people in the USA, is that the home is much more than a physical shelter. It becomes 'the most powerful sign of the self of the inhabitant who dwells within' (p. 123). They quote one respondent who replied 'I'd say my home is my castle. Even more than that, I'd say that home is church to me . . . to find peace and quiet and beauty with no static . . .' (p. 123).

For Ratty Tyler, the ageing farmworker in Angela Huth's *Land Girls*, one of his most valued possessions is the boxes of letters he keeps in the attic from his only son Edward who was killed in the First World War. The letters are more than a reminder of his son – they extend by association to represent the history of his marriage and the breakdown in communications with his shrewish wife Edith (Ratty and Edith are no Darby and Joan, the old couple of traditional storytelling who grow old together in devoted love and companionship). Ratty's view of his own self, now he is an old man, is bound up with the memory of his son:

> Ratty knew most of these letters by heart . . . sometimes he used to think Edward would be a writer when the war was over. He had the talent, surely. Ratty never mentioned this to Edith: she would have scoffed at so unmanly a suggestion. She probably had no idea the letters still existed. Unsentimental woman. Ratty had found her screwing up Edward's letters as she read them. If it hadn't been for Ratty's secret hoarding, there would be no voice, no words from Edward left.
>
> (Huth 1998: 87)

Ratty and Edith have been married for 51 years and the bundles of letters symbolize the tension that exists between them, as they live out their later lives united in a constant struggle.

In Paul Bailey's *At The Jerusalem*, Mrs Gadny is admitted to The Jerusalem, a workhouse converted by a reformed Victorian aristocrat into 'a home for the elderly and dying' (1987: 14). Mrs Gadny's personal mementos are now reduced to a small collection in a suitcase under her bed in the ward where she sleeps. It contains 'her choicest underwear, Tom's [her husband] Bible, some lavender in a cotton bag, a maid's cap and a pile of photographs' (p. 47). Photographs are, of course, often the most important reminders of our past lives and a fellow inmate, Mrs Capes, persuades Mrs Gadny to take them out so they can make comparisons. Mrs Capes keeps hers in a book which is covered in dust: ' "It hasn't seen daylight since I don't know how long. Like the best china, it only comes out on special occasions." She brought the book level with her chin and blew the dust off' (p. 48).

In what they describe to the nurse as 'a photo session' of exchanging memories (p. 55), the pair go in turn through their photographs identifying family members and reminiscing. But then a shocking event occurs when Mrs Gadny suddenly tires of the exercise and begins to tear up her own photographs. The nurse and Mrs Capes are outraged and can only conclude that Mrs Gadny is deranged. In her own mind, however, her motives are crystal clear:

Mrs Gadny screamed 'Don't touch me!' She was delighted she sounded so ferocious. 'Don't touch!'

They let her go.

'Mrs Gadny —'

'Your photos —'

'I don't need them. What use are they?'

'Reminders —'

'Souvenirs —'

'To stir memories —'

'I don't need them.' She added, serenely: 'I have their faces in my head. I have no use for photographs.'

(Bailey 1987: 57)

As readers we are aware that Mrs Gadny is extremely unhappy in The Jerusalem and she is reminded as she looks through the photographs that she is falsely complying with the official role expectation of the 'happy' and adjusted inmate. Whatever the sentimental value of her photographs she is prepared to sacrifice them in a more authentic personal statement. But the staff and other inmates are totally unable to understand this departure from the stereotypical well-adjusted role and the inevitable price Mrs Gadny pays is to be defined by them as a social deviant. From the matron's perspective Mrs Gadny's sudden action is irrational, a symptom of deeper psychological problems. She is no longer a 'normal' old woman satisfied, with her small collection of memories, to sit out the end of her days in smiling compliance. Eventually Mrs Gadny is labelled a madwoman and locked in a room on her own. The privacy she craves is ironically delivered in the form of a sentence to solitary confinement.

Places and spaces

Because places provide the material and symbolic framework for the cultivation of personal selves, they make an essential contribution to the construction of the age identity of the residents and are therefore a useful resource for writers of fiction. The identification of someone as old is shaped by the location in which they are encountered.

The reflexive interaction between place and selfhood is illustrated in Marika Cobbold's second novel, *A Rival Creation* when Evelyn Brooke, a doughty nature conservationist with a flourishing natural garden ages almost overnight when it is vandalized by a vengeful neighbour. For Miss Brooke's garden is the complete external expression of her inner self and she is speedily transformed from the formidable Evelyn Brooke into a pathetic old woman. ' "Old Miss Brooke", Liberty repeated sadly to herself. . . . It was no longer splendidly "Bloody Evelyn", or "that menace", let alone "the owner of that wonderful garden". No, it was "old Miss Brooke", and that Liberty thought, was truly the end' (p. 248). The passion that had kept Evelyn's garden going had been destroyed and she assumes the appearance and manner stereotypically associated with ageing. Her figure becomes 'hunched', she displays a 'defeated' look on her face (p. 282); she begins to speak constantly about her age, and appears to be suffering from lapses of memory. Liberty, who is 39, sadly remembers Evelyn 'had taught her that it was not being old that made you pitiful, only talking about wanting to be younger, as if that was all you wanted to be in your life. No, the trick was to behave as if you were completely at ease with your age, and everyone else would be too' (p. 281).

'Emplacement', as it is described in the sociology of ageing, is linked to age identity: there is, as Glenda Laws has observed, a 'complicity between body and landscape, embodiment and emplacement, in the creation of identity' (1997: 254). This is clearly reflected in the view that older people should be located in the particular places deemed appropriate to their age and circumstances. Society, as Goffman famously observed, 'establishes the means of categorising persons and the complement of attributes felt to be ordinary and natural for members of each of these categories' (1968: 11). To be out of place is to lay oneself open to possible criticism or even moral condemnation. Laws has noted the implications for age categorization: 'The material spaces and places in which we live, work and engage in leisure activities are age-graded and, in turn, age is associated with particular places and spaces' (1997: 90–1). In Barbara Pym's novel *A Few Green Leaves* the older people (women) in the village can be most easily encountered as a group gathered in the doctor's surgery. And Sam Martin, who has deliberately chosen to retire to a seaside village in Stanley Middleton's *Necessary Ends* repeatedly comments on the marginalization of older people – a marginalization indicated by the space one occupies.

Generally speaking, we expect to find older people is specific locations. And these locations become identified with the process of ageing as such. People spread out into places. Leder (1990) speaks of the 'extended body' (pp. 34–5) by which he means the process through which the body extends into the house: the walls of the house 'form a second protective skin, windows acting as artificial senses, entire rooms, like the bedroom or kitchen, devoted to a single bodily function' (p. 34). When he returns from holiday to find his house has burnt down David Renwick's Victor Meldrew in *One Foot in The Grave* pokes gloomily around in the ashes of what had once been home for him and Margaret for most of their married lives: 'Home. It had been that for more years than he liked to remember. It had been the Universe. It had clothed the two of them like a second skin, it had been their dearest friend. It had been the cocoon in which they had both developed, matured and ultimately begun to rot' (Renwick 1992: 76).

Perhaps the classic and most familiar fictional description of the association between a run-down house and its ageing occupant is found in Charles Dickens' *Great Expectations*. There is a close correspondence between descriptions of Miss Havisham's house – 'of old brick and dismal' with 'a great many iron bars to it' and several 'walled up' windows (1985: 84) – and Miss Havisham, the reclusive, prematurely aged woman, living out an embittered existence in curtained rooms among the decaying remains of her wedding feast. Jilted by her husband to be, her life and the life of the house are in deep decline: all the clocks have been stopped at 'twenty minutes to nine' (p. 88), the moment when her heart was broken.

An example of an old house as symbolic of the synchronized ageing of persons and their places occurs in James Long's *Ferney*. A young married couple, Mike and Gally, are looking for a house to buy in Somerset. They visit Mrs Mullard whose cottage may be for sale. The cottage, like Mrs Mullard, is stereotypically ramshackle:

> flanked by disintegrating outbuildings in paddocks fenced by rusty chicken wire. Mrs Mullard was an old vixen, an English gentlewoman gone wild, as gnarled as a briar root. . . .
> 'Come in and sit down,' said the old lady. She would not have been much over five foot two if she stood straight, and her arched spine lopped a further four inches off that. The room into which she led them had its parched floorboards half-covered in irregular patches of lino. She settled herself into the one complete article of furniture, a cracked brown leather armchair, and smiled questioningly while Mike and Gally perched on the unpadded frame of an old sofa.
>
> (Long 1998: 24)

In R.C. Sherriff's *The Fortnight in September*, first published in 1931, Mr and Mrs Stevens, who live in London, have taken their family for the last 20 years for a fortnight's holiday at the Huggett's boarding house, Seaview, in Bognor on the south coast. This is an established family tradition but the Stevens now become aware of the gradual change in Mr and Mrs Huggett and Seaview which has taken place over the years:

> Mr Huggett, originally blooming like a ripe plum – had begun to shrink. His crimson cheeks began to fade – leaving a network of tiny purple veins. One September the Stevens had noticed how thin his hands had become, how the skin sagged round the knuckles, and how his hand had shaken as he signed the receipt.
>
> (Sherriff 1974: 9–10)

The physical changes the Stevens observe in the Huggetts are closely interwoven with the decline of their business as former clients begin to cancel reservations and their future becomes insecure. The Stevens, who are loyal to Seaview, also recognize that the place is, like its owners, becoming out of date.

At the end of the novel Mrs Stevens has a disturbing encounter with Mrs Huggett (Flossie) who is clearly strained and nervous. When Mrs Huggett unexpectedly confides her fear that the boarding house is losing its attraction for holidaymakers Mrs Stevens experiences a 'queer feeling' she can't explain: 'It was as if one wall of "Seaview" had suddenly crumbled to the ground' (Sherriff 1974: 297). She is forced to confront the fact that the Huggetts and Seaview are ageing in tandem; they are becoming old-fashioned and their former guests are looking for more modern holiday accommodation. And by implication the Stevens, loyal to Seaview for 20 years, are growing older with them. ' "You see the real trouble" ', says Mr Stevens, ' "It isn't comfortable here, any longer – for people who don't understand. We've got to look things in the face, Flossie. Those old chairs downstairs – and this bed. We understand, but some people don't . . ." ' (p. 299). Out of compassionate loyalty the

Stevens decide to stay on an extra day to make a small compensation to the Huggetts for their loss.

The conventional idea of the 'look of age' often requires the establishment of significant points of similarity between older people, decaying material objects and buildings or parts of buildings. In Agatha Christie's *Sleeping Murder* an older man is compared with a 'house with its blinds pulled down' (1994b: 192–3). In the same story we can compare the house of Mr Galbraith who lives in Calcutta Lodge (echoes of an imperial past: Galbraith was in business in Calcutta in the 1920s), with the home of the humbler country couple Lily Kimble and her husband Jim. Calcutta Lodge is 'surrounded by a neat trim garden', and the sitting room is 'neat if slightly overcrowded', smelling 'of beeswax and Ronuk', with 'shining brasses.' (pp. 52–3). Galbraith himself is found sitting in his study. In contrast, Mrs Kimble and her husband are described in their kitchen where she is frying chips, an old newspaper spread on the table. In keeping with her lower social status she is 'Humming tune-lessly a popular melody of the day' while Jim, 'an elderly man of few words, was washing in the scullery sink' (p. 101).

In Peter Robinson's *Gallows View* a burglar distinguishes the homes of younger from those of older people: 'The old folks' houses all smelled of the past: lavender water, Vicks chest rub, commodes, old dead skin' (p. 38). And when an old lady, Alice Matlock, is found murdered in her home, the scene of the crime is described by Jenny, a young professor of psychology who is being consulted by the police, as 'oppressive':

> Not just because of the all-pervading presence of death, but because it was absolutely cluttered with the past. The walls seemed unusually hon-eycombed with little alcoves, nooks and crannies where painted Easter eggs and silver teaspoons from Rhyll or Morecombe nestled alongside old snuff boxes, delicate china figurines, a ship in a bottle, yellowed birth-day cards and miniatures. The mantelpiece was littered with sepia photo-graphs: family groups, stiff and formal before the camera, four women in nurses' uniforms standing in front of an old-fashioned army ambu-lance; and the remaining wall space seemed taken up by framed samplers, and watercolours of wildflowers, birds and butterflies. Jenny shuddered. Her own house, though structurally old, was sparse and modern inside. It would drive her crazy to live in a mausoleum like this.
>
> (Robinson 1988: 39–40)

Two negative aspects of the interpretation of ageing as decline are signifi-cant here. First, the idea that old age in particular has an unpleasant odour: the smell of disease, decay, and impending death (Corbin 1986). The power of the odours associated with disease and ageing to cause disgust has become so great that we attempt to segregate sick and older people from everyday living areas in the home when we confine them to the sickroom or remove them completely from the home into hospital and geriatric wards (Elias 1985; Bailin 1994). Second, the identification of the décor and furnishings of the homes of older people with the 'clutter' of the old fashioned past, which we noticed in the excerpts from Sherriff's *The Fortnight in September*. There, Mr and Mrs Stevens detect a close link between Mr and Mrs Huggett's physical decline and the fact that they are beginning to lose holiday bookings for their seaside boarding house because it is looking increasingly faded and out of date.

The Stevens are not deterred by the signs of the old fashioned because they provide a comforting assurance of the continuity of their own lives which is, of course, the reason that Mrs Stevens feels threatened. It is members of the younger generation who wish to break away from this link with the past. In Taylor's *A View of the Harbour*, a younger character, Lily Wilson compares the old town unfavourably with the new in the fishing village seaside resort where she lives. She sees the objects in the shop windows of the old town as 'symbols of the vanished life' (1995: 31–2): the 'strings of faded postcards' in the tobacconists, 'the Presents from Newby, the bald china head, mapped out and numbered in the palmist's window' (p. 32) can only be of interest to older people. The only people who appreciate the old town, says another character, Iris, during a discussion about the 'picturesque' quality of the place, are those who like old places and they are usually 'peculiar old fogies themselves' (p. 141).

The objects in the room of Sister Morris, who runs the residential accommodation Cherryfield in Cobbold's *Guppies For Tea*, appear to be designed to help her to dissociate herself from her clients:

> On the mantelpiece stood a collection of china pigs dressed in the manner of different professions. . . . Sister Morris herself shared her armchair with a large teddy, a calico cat and a giant, stuffed hedgehog, and on the coffee table stood an open Paddington Bear biscuit tin. She seemed determined to keep at bay the ever-present spectre of old age by cramming her tiny sitting room with childish whimsy.
>
> (Cobbold 1993: 105)

The displeasing smell of age is graphically captured in Susan Hill's *The Service of Clouds* when Molloy, the doctor who cares for older dying patients, enters the hospital: 'When he opened the doors into the hospital, the smell of it drowned him, the smell he had known as the background to his life, every day, every day – scrubbed sluices and antiseptic floors, sheets and sick bowls and the rank stems of flowers, and sweet, faecal decay' (Hill 1999: 5). In this all-to-familiarly depressing passage we are reminded again of Leder's (1990) dys-appearing body. Similarly, in Barbara Ewing's *The Actresses*, Harry, who is planning ahead for his retirement, makes his first visit to Copperfield House, a home for retired actors. He notices with distaste the smell of disinfectant mixed with another, slightly sour, smell pervading the theatrical surroundings of red carpet and ornate pictures of past members of the acting profession (1997: 91). The possibility that the ageing body will break out of its boundaries and cause offence appears almost impossible to conceal (Lawton 1998).

The places associated with ageing can be interpreted either positively or negatively and are influenced by distinctions of social class and status. The living conditions of the disadvantaged (and much larger) section of the older population in Britain are implied in incidental passages in Philip Caveney's thriller *Skin Flicks*. Danny Weston, the central character in the novel and a

32-year-old freelance photographer, visits his mother in her council flat in Manchester and we see through his eyes the physical surroundings in which she lives. They go into the 'malodorous little cubby hole that was her kitchen' to make a cup of tea:

> It wasn't her fault, she did her level best to keep it clean, but mainten-ance on these council-owned properties was little more than a rumour. Damp, rot and poor workmanship had taken their inevitable toll since Dad's death. He'd been a keen handyman, able to take all but the most serious problems in his stride.
>
> (Caveney 1995: 172–3)

Later Danny persuades his mother to allow him to take some photographs of her as she 'naturally is' in the old clothes she wears for sitting around the house. He takes several close-ups and experiences a sense of guilt when he finds himself in the depersonalizing role of photographer, treating his mother aesthetically as a kind of 'object framed in my shutter, something composed of lines and shadows and reflected light' (p. 176).

Class differences are central to accounts of places where people age in a number of novels by Pat Barker, who also pays close attention to gender differ-ences between the lives of working-class men and women. In these novels there is stringent and brilliantly observed commentary on the gender differ-ences that have been socially elaborated around the biological function of childbearing – the fact that it is women who conceive, carry and bear children. The capacity for motherhood is therefore integral to the perceptions of differ-ences in ageing between men and women. In *The Century's Daughter* memories of childbearing and rearing are central to the subjective world of the main character, Liza Jarrett, whom readers first encounter when she is an old woman in the 1980s. In her house, which hangs on as a dingy reminder of the past in an area surrounded by demolition, Liza struggles on with her box of memories. Her past life is reconstructed from her perspective through a series of flashbacks allowing the author to imaginatively recreate the history of working-class life in the North-east of England. But there is an additional per-spective on Liza's life: that of Stephen, the young homosexual social worker who visits her. A trusting relationship emerges which is supportive of Liza and influential on Stephen's life. Barker paints a grim, yet deeply humane picture of working-class ageing far from merely 'picturesque' efforts to find some aes-thetic value in the lives of poorer people and the places they inhabit.

The Victorian art critic John Ruskin was also fully aware of the fact that the visual appeal of picturesque paintings of aged labourers and slum dwellers was paid for in a high price of human suffering. And there is a danger in looking for aesthetic value or visual pleasure in the 'patina of age' in build-ings, on old stones and ageing as displayed in the 'natural' landscape where the effects of weathering or 'pleasing decay' extend to 'picturesque' old people (Lowenthal 1986: 164).

A contemporary version of the tension between the aesthetic valuation of ageing and an appreciation of the human costs incurred by the *effects* of social class on ageing occurs as we have seen when Danny Weston photographs his ageing mother. Weston is particularly well-placed to appreciate the significance of the dilemma because he specializes in taking pictures of older people, comparing them with decaying buildings. He has developed an aesthetic of ageing, little concerned with 'capturing the conventionally beautiful', and with a preference for 'the angular, the grotesque, the misshapen' (Caveney 1995: 8). He compares a yellow fungus growing on a blackened wooden beam in a rotting building with 'ancient skin, whorled and lined as if by passing years' and is reminded of a portrait he had made of a lady aged 94 'with some weird polyps growing on her cheek' (p. 12). His taste is for taking photographs of older people and drawing parallels between their external appearance and close-ups of the decay of the fabric of older buildings: brickwork, wooden beams and rusting metalwork.

There could hardly be a sharper contrast between these images of older places and people and those found for the most part in James Herriot's short stories based upon his life as a vet in North Yorkshire. Although they share in common an awareness of the interdependence of self and place, his images of ageing offer a less harrowing interpretation of the effects on the ageing process of the rigours of a life of hard labour. In his portrayals of country life (a mixture of factual observation and sympathetic imagination) resilient, dignified and sturdy old people are frequently encountered. Graham Lord, Herriot's biographer, describes the ingredients that have made Herriot's work so popular: 'the charming descriptions of an extinct society and a lost way of life; the rugged, unforgettable characters living with their ancient ways on their remote farms; the smell of the moors' (1998: 194). In, for example, *If Only They Could Talk*, there are:

> deeply moving moments . . . like the tragic story of the tiny, poverty-stricken old widower who lives in a cold, dank hovel and whose last friend, a cross-bred labrador, is so riddled with cancer that James has to put it down. There is also social comment: describing the old man's poverty and the meagre meal on the table, Alf reminds the reader that this is how pensioners have to live because the state pension is so small.
>
> (Lord 1998: 195–6)

Herriot does not therefore fail to appreciate the fact that such older people are living in poverty-stricken circumstances but prefers, as someone who is deeply attracted to life in the Yorkshire Dales, to celebrate the moral and physical courage with which they face adversity.

Although it was first published in 1970, *If Only They Could Talk* is set in the years immediately before the Second World War. The opening paragraphs of the story of the impoverished widower and his ailing dog graphically describe the derelict location of the house tersely noted down on a slip of paper: 'Dean, 3, Thompson's Yard. Old dog ill' (Herriot 1973: 84). Once inside the house:

> The grim evidence of poverty was everywhere. In the worn out lino, the fireless hearth, the dank, musty smell of the place. The wallpaper hung away from the damp patches and on the table the old man's solitary dinner was laid; a fragment of bacon, a few fried potatoes and a cup of tea. This was life on the old age pension.
>
> (Herriot 1973: 85)

There is clearly a close affinity between the old man and the old dog, although Herriot has no choice but to put the terminally ill animal down. The pathos of the moment, reminiscent of a Victorian genre painting of a cottage-dweller and his faithful companion, is however rescued from ending in sentimentality when Herriot leaves the house, having refused any payment:

> I said goodbye and went out of the house, through the passage and into the street. In the bustle of people and the bright sunshine, I could still see only the stark, little room, the old man and his dead dog.
>
> As I walked towards my car, I heard a shout behind me. The old man was shuffling excitedly towards me in his slippers. His cheeks were streaked and wet, but he was smiling. In his hand he held a small, brown object.
>
> 'You've been very kind, sir. I've got something for you.' He held out the object and I looked at it. It was tattered but just recognizable as a precious relic of a bygone celebration.
>
> 'Go on, it's for you,' said the old man. 'Have a cigar.'
>
> (Herriot 1973: 88)

Resilience in the face of harsh life-and-death decisions also pervades Herriot's descriptions of happier encounters with older men and women during the course of his rounds. Here too the figures are usually described as integral with the landscape – hardy individuals deeply grounded in beautiful countryside shaped by relentless natural forces. One such is Mr Stokill, a character from *All Things Wise and Wonderful,* who calls Herriot out on a bitterly cold winter's day. As he drives up the Dale Herriot admires the mystery and excitement of the winter landscape but when he gets out of the car:

> The thrill I felt at the strange beauty was swept away . . . and the wind struck me. It was an Arctic blast screaming from the east, picking up extra degrees of cold as it drove over the frozen white surface. I was wearing a heavy overcoat and woollen gloves but the gust whipped its way right into my bones. I gasped and leaned my back against the car while I buttoned the coat up under my chin, then I struggled forward to where the gate shook and rattled. I fought it open and my feet crunched as I went through.
>
> (Herriot 1979: 70)

Mr Stokill is over 70 and Herriot finds him forking manure. The contrast is between Herriot as a young man, an outsider captivated by nature's wild beauty, and the older local who has struggled with recalcitrant nature all his life and is oblivious of the weather. Unlike the warmly wrapped vet, Stokill seems to wear little protection against the bitter cold: 'A light khaki smock fluttered over a ragged navy waistcoat, clearly once part of his best suit, and his shirt bore neither collar nor stud. The white stubble on his fleshless jaw was a reproach to my twenty-four years and suddenly I felt an inadequate city-bred softie' (Herriot 1979: 70).

The concluding paragraph of this story is a good example of the belief that a lifetimes's identification with a particular place can be a source of wisdom in later life (Mr Stokill has displayed a masterly skill in handling animals):

As I followed him into the little building I smiled to myself. This old man had once told me that he had left school when he was twelve, whereas I had spent most of the twenty-four years of my life in study. Yet when I looked back on the last hour or so I could come to only one conclusion. He knew a lot more than I did.

(Herriot 1979: 76)

The older people who appear in James Herriot's stories also include solitary figures like the old man and his dying dog, or like old Albert Close, a retired shepherd who sits in a village pub, the Fox and Hounds, 'in the same place every night at the end of the settle against the fire' with his retired sheepdog (1979: 112). In these examples, the character is not only identified as situated in a particular location but also in terms of a close interdependency of man and animal. The meaning of the ageing of these people is determined by the physical environment: embodied humanity is closely identified with the land.

These examples clearly show that the identification of older people with particular places and spaces is by no means entirely negative; sometimes – as in the case of the problematic aesthetic of ageing (the question of the 'picturesque') – it is highly ambiguous, and sometimes it is positively celebratory. As Herriot's work indicates there are real personal strengths to be derived from a sense of belonging and this conclusion can be more generally applied. In Kathleen Rowntree's *Mr Brightly's Evening Off* the fictitious Chedbury, a small market town in middle England, is described as 'the perfect place in which to spend one's declining years' (1997: 11).

The celebration of a location and sometimes the nostalgia that accompanies it are significant elements in the social construction of ageing. Location is an important factor in the success of Roy Clarke's long-running television comedy *Last of The Summer Wine* set, as Bernice Martin has noted, in 'an idyllic Yorkshire village which evokes nostalgic sentiments about moorland landscape, Englishness, and lost community' (1990: 47, quoted in Blaikie 1999: 167). In keeping with this affinity between people and places, Roy Clarke dedicates his novel, *Gala Week*, which concerns the antics of his three older men, Foggy, Clegg and Compo, to 'gentle spirits and peaceful places' (1987). Bill Owen, the actor who played Compo, the most mischievous of the three characters, describes the series in his autobiography as one where three 'middle-aged men, all out of work, spend their time together in a Yorkshire village, ambling around, talking, thinking up ways of occupying themselves, getting into trouble, having fun' (1995: 166). In an image of retirement which is far more light-hearted than Stanley Middleton's story of Sam Martin's life in a Norfolk village (*Necessary Ends*) or Percy's disillusioning experiences in the decaying seaside town of Sutton's *Gorleston*, Compo, Clegg and Foggy are like irrepressible schoolboys or as Owen described them, referring to Richmal Crompton's schoolboy hero Just William (Hepworth 1996), 'geriatric "Just Williams"' (1995: 190). However, it has to be said that their mental and physical agility removes them far from any images of decline with which the label 'geriatric' is commonly associated. Owen himself developed such an affinity with Holmfirth, the location where the series was recorded, that he made a home there: a feeling he described as *'knowing* I am at home in Holmfirth and where I will no doubt find a final resting place' (1995: 159). Holmfirth, he also observed, is now described in a Yorkshire guide book as 'The Summer Wine Town' (1995: 177). An example of the essential interaction between fiction and reality.

Novelists are often credited with putting people accurately in their places; of seeing them as part of the landscape, and writers work with their particular vision of landscape and places: Stanley Middleton's Nottingham, for example, is partly real and partly an imaginative creation, as is James Herriot's Yorkshire Dales. Fiction requires an 'interaction of place and emotion, of past and present, of reality and imagination' (Drabble 1979: 152). The hold of places over the imagination is neatly described in Susan Hill's *The Service of Clouds*. In the following passage, Molloy, an ageing doctor who devotes much of his time to the care of older dying patients in a run-down, decaying hospital, is portrayed as a man who has since his childhood been 'haunted by places':

> He dreamed not of people but of rooms, of hallways, porches, attics, of the curve of a pillar, the moulding of a ceiling, the grain of a wooden beam. Of bannisters, steps, window-frames. By day, some part of a building he had known would be thrown upon the inner screen of his mind, and he would gaze at it. Time and again he would find himself walking, in his imagination, up some particular staircase and through a once-familiar door.
>
> (Hill 1999: 27)

We usually think of people in terms of the places they inhabit or are located. In Susan Hill's novel the physical decay of the patients tended by Molloy corresponds with the state of decay of the hospital building. When the hospital has been cleared and left derelict: 'Molloy still walks the empty corridors in his mind, sleeping or waking, hears the moaning and stirring and sudden little cries of the old men and old women (dead now) and the rush of wind up the basement stairs, the hushing sound of the ward door as it closes' (Hill 1999: 108).

Location is closely linked through categorization to social identity (Hepworth and Featherstone 1974). Traditionally, 'grannies' are supposed to live in rose-covered cottages, old tramps sleep under hedgerows and in general individuals are identified by the places where they live. Many surnames are, after all, derived from the places of our forebears. Descriptions of characters often draw parallels between the external appearance of their location and themselves: 'Our model of the person, our model of ourselves, does not exist in isolation. Our model is always set in a landscape, the landscape of the world that we have constructed' (Rowe 1989: 44).

Places are contexts and resources. What Gubrium (1995) describes as 'locally shared resources' (p. 9) which include the people in a locality – 'mundane features of local image' people like ' "you and me" ' (p. 10) – and various local settings within which selves are shaped. In Stanley Middleton's *Necessary Ends* Sam Martin retires to a bungalow in a Norfolk village where a number of other retired people are already in residence. Here the social status of older people continues to be measured by housing. Some of the older people in the village, says Sam, live in houses 'far too large for their needs' because 'a house confers status. You can't have retired admirals living in poky cottages. They've got to cut a dash, however inconvenient to themselves' (1999: 158). Thus the social distinctions of a younger life continue to exercise their influence in later life. Serena Burley in Hegarty's *Let's Dance* is dementing in a large house with Corinthian columns but she is being looked after by her daughter and her son Robert is aware of her social advantages compared with 'a lot of other little old ladies' who have no 'modicum of health' and limited financial resources (1996: 132).

Earlier we noted the affinity that is often perceived to exist between ageing people and places and the social construction of this affinity in, for example, the aesthetic of the picturesque or what Lowenthal describes as the 'look of age' (1986: 125). Because this affinity is socially constructed rather than a spontaneous occurrence – the result of assuming that older people 'naturally' inhabit certain places – the assumption of a fit or close correspondence can be highly misleading, thus giving a writer a nice opportunity to play around with these stereotypes to mystify and mislead other characters in a novel and sometimes to spring surprises on the reader. A good example of this is Joanna Trollope's *The Men and the Girls*. Here Miss Beatrice Bachelor is at first sight a typical Oxford spinster. Her accommodation in a first-floor bedsitting room is tastelessly furnished, 'crammed' with late Victorian furniture ('heavy and overbearing') and 'cheerless'. Her carpeting is 'muddy, the sad curtains unlined' and 'only the walls relieved the ugliness, being covered with postcards and larger reproductions of the Italian works of art Miss Bachelor so loved' (1993: 42). Predictably Miss Bachelor offers her visitor 'very dull biscuits' from 'an octagonal tin patterned with vaguely oriental herons and peonies' (p. 41). But this first impression is a false one. Beneath this façade there is a highly individual, vigorous, stimulating and very practical older woman who is able to establish rapport with a difficult teenage girl and with the other characters in the novel. Miss Bachelor can thus lay claim to being one of contemporary fiction's positive images of ageing.

Louise Doughty, in *Honey-Dew*, is another writer who imaginatively manipulates the image of the spinster: in this case the character of Miss Crabbe, an older woman living in a cottage in the English countryside. Externally her house looks very similar to its twin next door but inside it departs from what the narrator, Alison, expects to find in the home of an older spinster because it is packed with books and newspapers: 'I thought that old ladies who lived alone were supposed to be incredibly clean and tidy and dust their vases every day. Not Miss Crabbe' (1998: 50). Miss Crabbe has a fondness for crime fiction and is writing a crime novel by hand in pencil. She is in the process of creating a character she calls Miss Hartington. Here is the shade of Miss Marple in an 83-year-old investigator who is engaged in a kind of masquerade of elderliness by deliberately cultivating the image of 'an elderly eccentric' in order to 'misbehave in the way that normally only children were allowed to' (p. 61). Her simulated eccentricity includes walking down to the village in her slippers. The point is, of course, that in 'normal' everyday life older women do not track down murderers.

It is very often the periodization of the furnishings and fittings in a home that provides an age-related 'backdrop' to the person living in the house: a peep into the past. Desmond, a long-distance coach driver who is searching for the young son he has never seen in Deborah Moggach's *Driving in The Dark*, calls on Mrs Selwyn who he hopes can help him in his search. Mrs Selwyn is an older woman living in sheltered accommodation and her sitting-room is described as follows:

> While she boiled the kettle I looked around the room. There were photos along the shelves, and a flowery armchair with that napkin thing on the back to stop your hair getting it greasy. In front of the fire lay an overfed cat. It was like stepping back into my past. She had the *Radio Times* and knitting on the table; I bet she had grandchildren.
>
> (Moggach 1989: 65–6)

Yet here again appearances are deceptive. Although the inside of Mrs Selwyn's home is conventionally grandmotherly, she surprises Desmond by asking for a cigarette and revealing her fondness for a bet on the horses. She mocks the assumption that older women such as herself have nothing to do but play the granny role and look after other people's children. In fiction the stereotypical trappings of age can be artfully manipulated to maintain the reader's interest in the identity of particular characters.

In Sackville-West's *All Passion Spent* the house is central to the story of the positive ageing of Lady Slane. At the age of 81 she leaves her aristocratic family home Elm Park Gardens in London on the death of her husband to move to the small house in Hampstead for which she has secretly yearned for 30 years. The move of place signifies a change of self – pleasing oneself in later life – and it is not only the decision to leave the family home that affronts her children but also her intention to live away from them in a house on her own. Her move is a declaration of independence by an older woman from the domestic sphere. Lady Slane has no intention of adopting the conventional grandmotherly role. The family, as representatives of conventional attitudes to aristocratic older widows, even go so far as describing her decision as 'mad' (p. 68); the idea of living alone (with one woman servant) is, says her son Herbert, 'impossible' (p. 63). She is, they accuse, 'going to become completely self-indulgent' and, significantly, 'to wallow in old age' (p. 67).

Ageing is for Lady Slane an opportunity to publicly express a self which is disconcertingly different from the role she has dutifully performed for most of her life. The surfacing of this dimension of her inner self into public view is also marked by her removal of several of the rings she has worn for years as gifts of affection from her husband but also 'proper to the hands of Lord Slane's wife' (p. 74). In the course of this symbolic act she regards her hands, 'loaded with rings' (p. 73), with detachment 'as though they belonged to another person' (p. 74) – that is, the Lady Slane of the past who is in the process of transforming herself into the Lady Slane of the future. She keeps only those rings she 'had worn so long that they had become a part of her' (p. 75) and hands the rest over to her son Herbert.

Changes in personal identity associated with the ageing process are publicly and symbolically accomplished through changes in our biographical objects and the places where we live. When in Doris Lessing's *Love Again* Sarah Durham has come to the end of her love affairs with younger men and her daughter phones to say she is bringing the children for Christmas, she imagines her flat 'through the eyes of sunny and unproblematic California' and throws out the contents she now sees as 'junk'. The painters are brought in and, like Lady Slane, she retains the objects she regards as close to herself: part of her 'emotional history'. Once this alteration has been made to her material surroundings Sarah feels 'as if a weight had been lifted away out of her rooms, leaving her lighter and freer too' (1996: 337).

Discarding objects, redecorating rooms and moving house are part of the process that Diane Vaughan (1988) has described in her symbolic inter-actionist study of divorce as 'uncoupling'. As Penelope Lively puts it in *City of the Mind*, when a marriage breaks up the home is 'dismantled' (1992: 52) and there is a 'parcelling out of objects' (p. 51). The ageing process can therefore be seen as a process of disengagement from others which is deliberately chosen by the individuals concerned rather than being imposed upon them by others. This voluntary aspect of identity change in later life is, of course, the reverse of the situation where older people wish to maintain existing relationships or to symbolically sustain interaction with close relations now dead: 'Older widows and widowers . . . may continue to enjoy significant social relationships with their "dead" spouse' and objects left behind such as clothing and photographs 'can bring the partners closer' (Hallam *et al.* 1999: 149).

Home

As we have seen from a number of the previously quoted excerpts from novels and from the comments of social analysts, the strongest formative influence of place on self – and certainly the most emotive – is the home. Nostalgia, a powerful emotion which is frequently associated with the experience of ageing, was originally defined as 'homesickness', but as we have also seen, attitudes to home may have a strongly ambivalent quality.

In Anita Brookner's *A Private View*, home for newly retired George Bland is a luxury flat in London. George has never married, has had a financially rewarding career, and makes forays out into the world – foreign holidays, visits to libraries, museums and art galleries – from 'the second floor of a handsome modern block in a quiet street equidistant from the park and the Edgeware Road' (1995: 18). But home, for all its comfort, is ambivalent. Although it is George's own choice – what he hoped would be 'his own creation', an expression of 'his own personality' – it is somehow unsatisfactory (p. 19) and he experiences his flat ambivalently as both a 'refuge' and a source of exasperation:

> Home is where the heart is. Alternatively, Home is so sad. Bland's attitude towards his flat was the somewhat shifting point at which these two attitudes conjoined. When he was away from it he thought of it longingly, as the place which would always provide him with a refuge from the world. When he was actually inside it, safe and warm and quiet, as

he had always wished to be, it exasperated him. . . . The quietness, which he cherished, tormented him.

(Brookner 1995: 18)

Whatever level of ambivalence we may feel towards home, when we are faced with the prospect of losing our home or when we have no home we become the object of pity. In Thea Astley's novel *Coda*, Kathleen is battling with her awareness of increasing confusion. Her friend, called Daisy, has only a few personal possessions left and lives in fear of someone breaking into her home and stealing them. Consequently, she carries them around with her. They are a few photographs, her pension bank book, her health card, and a book she won in primary school. When she is hit by a reversing truck these objects are pathetically scattered into the street, collected into a bag by passers-by and thrown away as rubbish.

The home is seen as the most appropriate place for older people and is defined in social gerontology as 'an essentially private place which is the centre of domesticity, a place of intimacy and sometimes a place of solitude' (Bond 1993: 204). Home is the place which is segregated from the public sphere – a place where the private self is cultivated, nurtured and expressed, and any consideration of the home inevitably involves some discussion of the influence of gender on ageing.

The division of labour which produced the separation of work from home during the nineteenth century transformed the home into what was regarded by many as the only appropriate place for women. The domestic sphere has therefore become a valuable resource for novelists because of the 'emotional and affective relations which women have with home-making' (Light 1991: 219). Domesticity can be interpreted as 'a complex knot of feelings, ideas and activities which have structured a sense of feminine self' (Light 1991: 219). The significant interconnection is the interaction between the internal or 'interiority' as Light calls it, and the external world. The social division of labour between men and women produces for women a domesticated self where 'housework . . . "home-making" and the acquiring of "things" . . . have played a . . . part in the dreams as well as the "oppression" of different women'. The sense of feminine self is structured through objects in the domestic sphere but the domestic sphere, Light warns, is not only about the tensions and divisions between women and men but also about tensions and divisions between women and women: 'The carpet and the three-piece suite, the hoover and the new gas-oven are icons of hope and dignity as well as pride and envy' (p. 219). Home-making is a process of physical and emotional effort, establishing and creating the self. Home-making is self-making. One author who has graphically and sensitively explored the effects of gender divisions and social and economic exploitation on the experiences of ageing among working-class women and men in the North of England is Pat Barker.

In the home the room set aside for containing the body in ill health is the sickroom. And in the sickroom it is often women who do the caring. Now that he is a chronic invalid Ike's room in Smiley's *At Paradise Gate* is separate from the bedroom of Anna his wife of many years and now carer. Anna maintains her domestic control through tireless effort over the cleanliness and order of the rest of the house but the sickness of Ike's body seems to have spread throughout his room and become imprinted on it:

> The wallpaper, once a rose and dove gray stripe, had darkened to charcoal and maroon. The arms of the stuffed chair had frayed and the door of the closet bulged ajar with coats and bathrobes and outmoded dresses. The little rug she had braided needed washing, and interspersed with his books were letters and papers and old bills.
>
> (Smiley 1995: 97)

A central feature of the home which is an enormous asset to novelists is its privacy. The home, especially the respectable home, provides a space for the novelist within which the self may be cultivated. The fact that it is concealed from public view and readers are never quite sure what they are going to find inside is, of course, a staple feature of crime and horror stories. Penetration of the private sphere of the home is central to the novel. But the home, as we have seen, is ambiguous – it can also be a prison. Old age, when allied to sickness and disability, can confine both men and women to the home and such older characters are a boon to crime writers for a number of reasons. First, the fact that they are confined to one place and may be mentally alert means that they notice things other less close observers miss in the external world they can see. They are aware of subtle changes in timetabling and of the comings and goings of neighbours and strangers. Second, they exploit the stereotypical assumption that older people who are housebound are also mentally confused or incapable of accurate perceptions. This can allow the tension in a story to be maintained while the investigator gradually becomes aware of the value of the evidence.

Ruth Rendell makes use of this device in her crime story *Simisola*, where key evidence is provided by an old man who is confined to his room in an upstairs flat, spending his time watching events in the street. Almost until the end the value of what he has seen is ignored simply because of assumptions about his age and competence.

Inspector Burden first catches sight of this witness when waiting for someone to answer the door of a house at which he is calling: 'for some reason he looked behind him, the way we do when we think we are being watched. On the opposite side of the street, in a 1900-ish house with a short front garden, someone was looking at him from an upstairs window. A face that looked as old as the house, crinkled, frowning, glaring' (Rendell 1995: 53). The owner of the face which, in an interesting reaction, Burden almost mistakes for a mask, is 93-year-old Percy Hammond who lives alone except for the service of meals-on-wheels and the attentions of the blind ground-floor flat tenant, a woman aged 80. Hammond's fixed position in front of the window and his mental alertness mean that he is an ideal witness: someone whose ability to make an accurate identification makes a valuable contribution to the solving of the murder of the woman in the house opposite. One reason why it is hard to credit his observations is that Chief Inspector Wexford, who visits Hammond, can scarcely credit that he is any longer human. His first sight of him sleeping in his chair by the upstairs window makes Wexford wonder what he looked like when he was young: 'There was nothing in that creased, pouchy, stretched, puckered face to indicate the lineaments of middle age, still less youth. It was scarcely human any more. Only the white, rosy-gummed dentures, displayed when he smiled, hinted at real teeth, lost fifty years before' (p. 173).

Places, like people, age and change. In Susan Hill's *The Service of Clouds* Molloy, the ageing doctor, thinks back to his boyhood and the smart new houses on the road to the sea. But now, he thinks, 'those houses have old, old people struggling on in too many big rooms, behind overgrown, unmanageable gardens. There is nothing brash and new there any more, only decay, and sadness for the bright past' (1999: 28). So close is the association between places and the self that letting things go is a sign of 'letting oneself go'. But, as Rory Williams' (1990) interviews with older men and women in Aberdeen show, there comes a time when submission to the decay of old age is considered socially acceptable after a period of honourable struggle with the illness and frailty of the body. Not letting things go is an indication of moral effort which should only be relinquished when a person is physically unable to carry on the upkeep of the house. To let things go is to pass into what Williams describes as 'a second stage of ageing' (p. 63), equivalent to Leder's (1990) dys-appearing body. For Williams' informants the physically diminishing effects of illness indicate the point of transition into 'true old age' (1990: 64): ageing is a moral struggle, as Jerrome (1992) observed, and there comes a point in the ageing process when individuals are no longer required to carry on the struggle against the effects of illness. It is illness which provides the final justification for 'seeing oneself as "really" old' (Williams 1990: 63). At this point surrender is honourable and one can then hope for bodily suffering to be terminated by a quick death.

In Laurie Lee's *Cider With Rosie*, a poetically sensitive memory of his childhood in a remote Cotswold village, there is a poignant description of final surrender in old age. First published in 1959, and described by him in an introductory note as a 'recollection of early boyhood' where 'some of the facts may be distorted by time', *Cider With Rosie* contains the memorable description of two older people: the apparently 'indestructible' Joseph and Hannah Brown. It was said, Lee recalls, that they had lived in their cottage by the common for 50 years, and he offers us a picture of two people so closely bound to the home that they cannot exist when removed from it:

> The old couple were as absorbed in themselves as lovers, content and self-contained; they never left the village or each other's company, they lived as snug as two podded chestnuts. By day blue smoke curled up from their chimney, at night the red windows glowed; the cottage, when we passed it, said 'Here live the Browns', as though that were part of nature.
>
> (Lee 1962: 109)

After a week or so when the Browns are not seen about, they are found in a sorry plight: Joseph collapsed on the floor and Hannah struggling to feed him. They are deemed no longer able to look after themselves by the 'authorities' and are taken into the 'care' of the workhouse. They plead to be allowed to stay outside the workhouse but in vain, and are separated for the first time for 50 years, dying within the week. 'Their cottage', writes Lee:

stood empty on the edge of the common, its front door locked and sound-less. Its stones grew rapidly cold and repellent with its life so suddenly withdrawn. In a year it fell down, first the roof, then the walls, and lay scattered in a tangle of briars. Its decay was so violent and overwhelm-ing, it was as though the old couple had wrecked it themselves.

(Lee 1962: 111)

Seen through the medium of Lee's creative imagination, the decay of the old couple goes in tandem with the place they inhabited. When they leave the cottage, almost like another human being it follows them into physical decline. In his narrative the old couple are not described in any detail but are realized in terms of the details of their home and its longevity: 'It seemed that the old Browns belonged for ever' (1962: 109).

Places and people, as Lowenthal (1986) has observed, are not static but subject to physical change. And the condition of changing rural life is where Lee's book leaves us: with the waning during the years between the First and Second World Wars of the world of childhood he knew: 'Time squared itself, and the village shrank, and distances crept nearer. . . . Old men in the pubs sang, "As I Walked Out", then walked out and never came back. Our Mother was grey now, and a shade more light-headed, talking of mansions she would never build' (1962: 230).

But the Browns' identity as a couple has survived their deaths in the decay-ing house and in Lee's writing, reminding us that identities may persist sym-bolically long after we are disembodied.

The transition from home to a 'home'

Although it may be regarded in professional circles as a sign of prudent prep-aration for the later part of life, an invitation to look around for a suitable place to live when one is no longer capable of looking after oneself is not always welcome. In Barbara Ewing's *The Actresses*, a novel about the fortunes of a group of middle-aged actresses and actors who were all members of the same drama class, Pauline is shocked to be informed that Henry has been looking around a home for retired actors. She sees his visit as a premature expression of anticipated ageing: ' "Strange," said Pauline. "I mean – thinking of being old like that when he's still young" ' (1997: 193). Mrs Beale, who runs Copperfield House, interprets Pauline's reaction as an indication of fear of 'old age and loneliness' (p. 194). In the same novel Harry, who is gay, pro-poses that he and Frances whose marriage is over, should buy a couple of flats and live side by side. ' "You mean",' says Francis, ' "grow old together?" '. But although she is very fond of Harry she rejects the idea: 'hidden in a very secret part of her mind was the vision of lonely ageing actresses at first nights and parties with gay men, the *fag hags* people called them, the animated chatter and waving and the loud loud smiles' (p. 356).

A similar proposal is made by Sarah Durham's middle-aged brother Hal whose marriage is on the verge of breaking up in Doris Lessing's *Love Again*. Like Francis she rejects the idea although for a somewhat different reason. She knows Hal is a totally self-centred man who is only capable of seeing a situation from his own point of view. He will demand her complete attention 'for the rest of her life' and 'was not seeing her even now' (1996: 321).

The move from the private home to a residential 'home' or to hospital, often described in the gerontological literature as a stressful transition in the ageing process (Hockey 1999a), is also a prominent narrative turning point in stories of ageing. In Simon Brett's murder mystery *A Nice Class of Corpse*, Mrs Pargeter goes to stay at the Devereux Hotel in Sussex, a private hotel for long-term guests from genteel backgrounds who are capable of living independent lives. It is run by Miss Naismith who speaks with a voice of 'daunting gentility' (1992b: 10) and who gathers around her a carefully selected group of genteel residents. The hotel is, Mrs Pargeter is informed by fellow resident Miss Wardstone, 'for *active* people. In other words, people who are physically fit and in full control of themselves' (1992b: 56). The result is that rivalries and tensions between residents are given a competitive edge and more drama is extracted to heighten the mystery. Ageing as a risk of loss of independence and institutionalization is a useful narrative device for the mystery story writer. Miss Naismith of the Devereux operates what residents refer to as the 'transfer list' (p. 56). This can be used as a threat and source of power both by the owner and by residents over each other. Miss Medlingham keeps a black notebook in which she records her efforts to remember names. One entry reads 'Getting names wrong is just the sort of thing Miss N. [the owner] notices and I don't want to give her any more ammunition. I must stay at the Devereux. I don't think I could cope with another move at my age' (p. 96).

The stress of making the transition from home to a 'home' is such that individual characters are sometimes described as having aged overnight when they enter hospital or care. After being physically attacked on a London street, Fanny Pye in Nina Bawden's *Family Money* is taken unconscious into hospital where she comes round to find she is no longer the independent individual she believed herself to be, but a dependent invalid who has memory loss. Fortunately this is a temporary problem and the rest of the novel shows Fanny finding her way back to full independence. Nina Bawden's novel is in this sense a story of positive ageing.

Anna in Jane Smiley's *At Paradise Gate* comes under pressure from her daughter Claire and granddaughter Christine to put the ailing Ike into hospital. Ike unexpectedly appears in the doorway 'frail but upright' and demands to know what they are 'whispering about' (1995: 134). Marika Cobbold's *Guppies For Tea* opens with Robert Merryman wheeling his mother Selma, against her will, into the Cherryfield home. Her room is to be 'Number Five, a small room, the shape of a shoe box, and the smell of disinfectant was stronger in spite of the open window at the far end'. It is sparsely furnished with a dressing table with an 'easy-to-clean' melamine top' and a chair under the window which Robert 'could not help thinking . . . you would never find in anyone's home' (1993: 12). Anxious, as many younger people are, to leave such a place, Robert tells Selma he must drive home: 'At the word home, Selma looked up, fixing him with eyes like pebbles, dulled by sand. She snatched his right hand back against her chest and held it there' (p. 13).

The negative effects of a change of place on the self of an older person – the move from home to a 'home' – are also described in reverse when Amelia, Selma's granddaughter, takes her out of Cherryfield to lunch with another resident, a retired admiral. Through Amelia's eyes we see how the change in situation produces a transformation in the older people: 'It was, Amelia thought, as if the atmosphere at Cherryfield was too thin to sustain real life and that now, back in the world, Selma and the Admiral filled out and coloured in, ceasing to be old people, and becoming just people' (Cobbold 1993: 54).

The 'home'

The most obvious site of age categorization is, of course, the residential 'home', popularly regarded as the appropriate setting for old age. But there are other collective settings for ageing, as we have seen above. In *At Bartram's Hotel* Agatha Christie collects a number of older people together in comparatively genteel suroundings for her crime story. Her idea is of a genteel hotel, a survival from a past Edwardian age, and a haven for older people in a backstreet of London's Mayfair, with the means for a luxuriously quiet life: 'Nice old-fashioned clientele, comfortable, old-fashioned premises, nothing rackety about it, a lot of luxury without looking luxurious' (1985: 126). When a man who is considerably younger than usual enters the reception area the hotel immediately takes on the 'atmosphere of a museum' and the guests appear to be 'the dust encrusted relics of a past age' (p. 26).

Miss Marple, who first stayed there 60 years before and revisits partly out of nostalgia, reflects on the cost of preserving an image of stability:

> She had never expected, not for a moment, that things would be as much like they used to be . . . because, after all, Time didn't stand still. . . . And to have made it stand still in this way must really have cost a lot of money. . . . Not a bit of plastic in the place! . . . it must pay them, she supposed. The out-of-date returns in due course as the picturesque. . . . None of this place seemed real at all. . . . Well, why should it? It was fifty – no, nearer sixty years since she had stayed here. And it didn't seem real to her because she was now acclimatised in this present year of our Lord . . .

> (Christie 1985: 36)

The fashion for making residential accommodation for older people the scene of crime has been satirized by Michael Dibdin in *The Dying of the Light*, which is set in an old people's home. Here a mixed cast of old residents are brought together in a seedy run-down old house, Eventide Lodge, where death is steadily reducing their number.

In residential homes for older people ageing is at first sight collectivized and correspondingly stereotyped. All the people are there because they all have similar problems caused by ageing. The administrative preoccupation with old age leads to the risk of losing sight of the individuality of older people and writers can draw on this aspect of the collective care of older people in two ways. They can construct stories which highlight the diversity of personalities and variations in social background or they can engage the reader with descriptions of the struggles of a central character to survive the negative pressures of institutionalization.

For the novelist one of the interesting features of residential accommodation is therefore the way in which it brings different categories of individuals into a social institution. People who have spent their lives maintaining their own private sphere – 'keeping themselves to themselves' – may be brought together into enforced socialization. Priory Lodge, the main location of Conlon's *Face Values* on the Lancashire coast – ' "geriatrica-on-sea" the bus driver called it' (1986: 9) – is a home for 'active elderly gentlefolk'. Elsa, aged 31, who has taken a job there, considers ageing to be 'a depressingly democratic process, not one whit kinder to Mrs Cuthbert-Carew or Mrs Booth-Powell than it was to the three ex-mill workers from Bradford enjoying their once-a-year breath of ozone' (p. 56). But in the same story there are descriptions of the lingering influence of social distinctions, impressed in the body of the residents and in their attitudes and actions. These are indicated, for example, in the inventory Elsa makes of the residents of Priory Lodge after her arrival when she is given a list of their names:

> She rehearsed each of the names again, adding rudimentary descriptions as an aide-memoire: first floor: Colonel Pritchard (tall, clean, mottled – kippers), Mrs Cuthbert-Carew (gnarled, aristocratic – grapefruit), Miss Vyner (arthritic, ex-Ministry of Works – All-Bran), Mrs Peglar (rich vulgar – bacon and egg and tomatoes), Mrs Booth-Powell – pronounced Po-elle (rich posh – poached egg), Mrs Pendennis (lovely bones, still good-looking, must have been a stunner in her day – Ryvita), second floor: Mrs Bannerman (a grey Buddha – toast and marmalade), Mrs Crookthorne (weasel-faced – eats everything going), Miss Johns (spinster, timid – porridge), Mrs Grey (widow, timid – muesli), Messrs Gentile (Italian, scarcely bilingual – porridge) and Golding (eyes Everywhere – and hands too – sausages).
>
> (Conlon 1986: 15)

This list indicates a potentially rich blend of diverse individuals and one of the risks of residential accommodation is that of being brought into unwelcome contact with undesirable and even dangerous older people. The satirical edge of Christopher Hope's *Serenity House*, a private home in North London, is that serenity is one of the last of the alleged benefits of later life experienced by the residents. Serenity House is run by Cledwyn Fox – ' "Remember this isn't *my* home, it's *yours*" ' (1993: 5) – who provides what appears to be a closely regulated and supportive environment. But the main character is Max Montfalcon, an individual Cledwyn Fox would once have

> called 'a gentleman', with his fine good grey hair carefully swept back over the ears, and his light blue eyes, even now with a tendency to water, still imposing and rather beautiful. His height and bearing, at eighty-one, made Max Montfalcon a handsome man, with his rather sad little habits – the elderly red tin of rolling tobacco in his inside pocket, shreds of the stuff lodging in the folds of his clothes and often in the folds of his facial skin, the distressing habit of walking with his heels flat, refusing to lace

his shoes properly and turning left and right foot sideways as he shuffled along, walking on his feet but not in his shoes. How he kept them on was a mystery. Yet he never lost a shoe, did Max Montfalcon, even when he went on one of his little 'wanderings' and had to be brought back from the park or the woods, or the heath where he'd been found like some stray dog or picked up like a lost ball.

(Hope 1993: 12)

Yet Cledwyn Fox also recognizes that this is a surface image: 'that what Max showed of himself was never the whole picture' (p. 61). Behind this crumbling façade Max lives out a nightmarish mental life populated by the memories of the number of people he killed in his secret past life in Hitler's Germany. In the pursuit of Nazi racial purity, his job was to help select out those who were considered worth keeping alive; separating the young from the old: 'old ones were sent away. It might take no more than five minutes. That was all, at the ramp. Someone nodded. "You left, you right" ' (p. 174). Ironically, of course, Max now lives in an institution dedicated to keeping those who have become mentally and physically frail – who 'really weren't up to it any longer' – alive (p. 11).

When a home for older people provides a private room it can be a haven for the cultivation of a secret life. Miss Primple, the resident who has stayed longest at The Hollyhocks in Bernice Rubens' *The Waiting Game* and whose public appearances are characterized for the most part by silence, spends most of her time in her room. Here we have an example of the cultivation of multiple selves for Miss Primple's public reticence is in sharp contrast with her private volubility. She has subscribed to her own private telephone line and is absorbed in anonymous conversations on chat lines which provide opportunities for 'double entendre' and 'innuendo' (1997: 44). Miss Primple's devotion of her later life to conversations with total strangers is a neat and ironic example of symbolic interaction: 'With her little hobby she had no need of fleshly company. No need of the tedious and repetitive talk of the old codgers in the downstairs lounge. No need to listen to their groans and their moans, their ill-concealed malice and bigotry (p. 44).

The private phone line is an escape route for Miss Primple from a boring situation. It provides a resource for playing out any number of roles including those of younger women, and for switching gender. Miss Primple has plenty of money to spend on calls and the range of multiple selves open to her is extensive. She is fully aware 'that to spend it in this fashion served sensibly to enhance the life quality of her remaining years' (p. 44).

One source of danger in a residential home may arise when certain residents, like Mrs Gadny in Bailey's *At The Jerusalem* no longer blend imperceptibly into the surroundings and, as we have seen, begin to act 'out of character'. Bernice Rubens has another vivid example in *The Waiting Game* when Miss Jennifer Bellamy, aged 80, who has hitherto been as quiet as a mouse, suddenly clutches the Christmas tree and grabs at a plastic figure of the baby Jesus:

'Fuck you,' she screamed at the plastic. Then turning to her astonished audience, 'And fuck you too. All of you. Fuck, fuck, fuck,' and a rogue tone of joy crept into her voice as she cursed them with a word, repeated over and over again, a word which she had never in her life used before, and of whose meaning she certainly had never had experience.

(Rubens 1997: 45)

Yet from the perspective of the onlookers, unexpected behaviour can come as an invigorating change, especially to people whose lives are monotonously routinized. The residents of The Hollyhocks who witness this episode are cheered by the failure of Miss Bellamy to keep up appearances and 'it promised to be a merry Christmas after all' (p. 46).

Social hierarchies are a source of rich material for authors writing stories about life in residential accommodation. As groups of older people gathered together under the same roof, residential homes offer a rich opportunity for the writer of imaginative fiction to create rivalries and tensions out of their everyday relationships. As such they offer plenty of scope for pathos and tragedy, but they are also places for the tragi-comic – as in Bernice Rubens' *The Waiting Game*. The Hollyhocks Home for the Aged is no ordinary home but a private home for which the matron selects only high-class residents. Within it is found a social hierarchy presided over by Lady Celia Suckling and the residents include Jeremy Cross, aged 79, 'a professional survivor' who has pinned to his wardrobe door a list of the names of the contemporaries he has outlived. His tragedy is that having survived one heart attack in the home he returns to experience a final one and his last emotions are provoked by his anger and loathing that others will outlast him. Suddenly he loses his ability to speak, his mouth moves but he can't hear any sounds:

On discharge from the hospital, he had been given a clean bill of health. Yet he slumped to the floor, astonished. Then the sounds came back, matching his mouth's movements.

'No!' he shouted. 'Absolutely no!' He was by no means the last bottle on the wall. He stared at Lady Celia with loathing. 'It's not fair,' he whimpered. 'You're older than me.' Then the pain seized him and, fair or not, he resigned from the waiting game.

(Rubens 1997: 206)

Jeremy Cross's dys-appearing body has taken him out.

5

Vulnerability and risk

Vulnerability in later life is associated with risk and danger. The dys-appearing body brings the risk of reduced independence and in certain respects the external world becomes more dangerous largely because it is not tailored to the requirements of people who do not correspond to the cultural ideal of youthfully active individualism. In this chapter we look at fictional representations of physical and mental vulnerability in later life and also at some of the dangers associated with specific places and the threat they pose to the integrity of the sense of self. We also look at alternative examples of older people who are still sufficiently powerful to act threateningly towards others – that is, at the idea of older characters themselves as risky and dangerous.

The thread of symbolic interactionism continues to weave its way throughout this narrative as we explore the ways in which fictional examples of the risks and dangers of ageing display variations in the essential interdependency of body, self and society.

Physical vulnerability

Ageing is a risky business. In particular, reports of the physical vulnerability of older people to attack in the news media are calculated to provoke pity and horror. The fear of physical attack among older people is a contentious issue but there is no doubt that a widespread perception exists that older people are particularly at risk. In John Harvey's *Easy Meat*, Eric and Doris Netherfield live in an area plagued by burglaries and for 12 years Eric has kept an iron railing within reach when they go to bed: 'the last thing Eric had done each night, after dropping his teeth into the glass beside the bed and wishing Doris God bless and good-night, was trail his fingers down towards that piece of iron, as if touching it for good luck' (1996: 53).

On one occasion his foresight is tested to the full when Nicky, a juvenile delinquent looking for easy money, breaks into the house. Eric, who has heard a creaking on the stairs, attacks Nicky first with the iron bar but is not strong enough to withstand Nicky's surprised rage. In a violent outburst – 'in the mirror, he caught a glimpse of his reflection, white and scared. Stupid cunt! What'd he have to have a go at him for? Why didn't he just let him run?' (p. 55) – Nicky grabs hold of the bar and savagely rains blows on the now defenceless couple 'until his arms had begun to ache and he had had enough' (p. 55). Inevitably the crime arouses the horror and disgust that follows disclosure of an unequal struggle and in this example we see the outcome of inequalities in the comparative physical strength of youth and age even when the latter is prepared and strikes first.

An additional source of anxiety is the knowledge that as 'shells of the self' and havens in a 'heartless world' homes are not impregnable but vulnerable to the invasion of strangers. Once their defences have been breached, Eric and Doris are quickly transformed into objects of pity and terror – the victims of violent physical attack whose battered faces occasionally appear in dramatic newspaper headlines and on TV screens. The anxiety associated with ageing in general is thus further specifically amplified as the external world is portrayed as potentially threatening to older people.

It is not, as we have seen, that older people make no resistance to violence or are incapable of violence but that their physical weakness transforms them into objects of pity and anger. Liza Jarrett, the central character in Pat Barker's *The Century's Daughter*, is violently attacked in her home by three delinquents who believe that money is concealed in the tin box of memorabilia she keeps under her bed. Liza, a working-class woman whose life course parallels the history of the twentieth century, and whose life story is the subject of the novel, is a spirited and valiant woman but she has at the end of her life been reduced by ageing and illness and a blow to her jaw from one of the frustrated intruders hastens her death. The pathos of the attack is accentuated by the fact that Liza has nothing of material value worth stealing. However, her social worker Stephen remembers after her violent death:

> 'She let too many people see that box. She was always dipping into it and pushing it under the bed. The result was they all thought she had money. I don't know where they thought she got it from. I used to go and get her pension and do her shopping for her and I can tell you there was bugger-all left by the end of the week.'
>
> (Barker 1986: 278)

This incident occurs at the end of the book and the reader's sense of outrage is intensified by the preceding narration of Liza's character and the moving story of her courageous lifelong struggle to maintain her personal dignity and independence in an industrial town in the North-East of England. Familiarity with the story of Liza's life means that readers are not allowed to see her stereotypically as just another old woman in a decaying post-industrial neighbourhood. She is a fully-rounded human being whose latter-day physical frailty deserves respectful care. Outrage is further intensified by the knowledge that her attackers are part of the neighbourhood network; the sons of local people.

Although ageing can expose older people to the risk of invasion and attack not all, as we have seen, are intimidated and some are well able to take the offensive. Stanley Middleton's *Live and Learn* opens with the pursuit of Jonathan Winter by four would-be muggers into a cul-de-sac. Winter, who is on his way home from a rugby club meeting, teaches at a university in the English Midlands. But although he is physically fit and in his twenties, he is outnumbered and wisely decides to run. Fortunately he is saved in the nick of time by a much older man who takes him into his house where he hides until the danger has passed. Once safely inside, Winter's rescuer shows him a loaded shotgun:

> The host, who had not yet sat down, marched from the room into the corridor and returned carrying a shotgun. It looked to Winter's unculti-vated eye to be clean, oiled, ready for use, exceptionally nasty.
> 'This is what I keep to welcome them.'
> 'Is it loaded?'
> 'It is.'
> 'Isn't that dangerous? You hear of such accidents.'
> 'You hear of accidents with carving knives, but I still keep one.'
> 'You would have used it?'
> 'If they had tried to force their way in.'
> 'Would it do much damage?'
> 'I'll say it would. Could kill. But there were four of them on to two of us. And I'm elderly. And you were there as a witness. An ideal oppor-tunity to use.' He patted the butt.
>
> (Middleton 1996: 3–4)

Once back in his own home, Jonathan reflects on the encounter and specu-lates about the older man's age and his preparations for self-defence:

> How old was he? Middle-fifties, perhaps? Educated voice. Decent furni-ture. One of two interesting pictures on his walls. Deep, colourful, newish carpets. But ready for invaders, Hookes had placed a loaded gun in the hall. Why was he at the front gate as Jonathan passed? Was he on the look-out for trouble? Did he actively court it? That was unlikely on a quiet side-street. Yet first time out, in shirt sleeves on a frosty night, he'd netted a fugitive. 'Keep on the path,' he'd warned. Had he lined his garden with mines or man-traps? It all seemed unlikely, and Jonathan grinned at his fancies.
>
> (Middleton 1996: 5–6)

In this story both younger and older people are represented as vulnerable to physical attack in certain places and at certain times. The inner city is a potentially dangerous place for both generations. But the incident also rein-forces the commonly held belief in the specific vulnerability of older people simply because they are physically weaker and must therefore make special preparations for the protection of self and property.

Hookes, like the less fortunate Eric Netherfield in John Harvey's *Easy Meat*, has armed himself against the invasion of his home and is also prepared for the possibility of attack on the city streets. From the perspective of older people city streets are often described as turbulent, disturbing and potentially threatening. In Thea Astley's *Coda*, set in Australia, Kathleen, who is becoming confused, is walking the city streets:

> slowly back to the Queen Street walking-place, a madhouse of tent-topped eateries and truant schoolkids rampaging past shop fronts. She was buffetted by racing hoons on roller blades and shoving teenagers, rendered invisible to them by her very age. Someone snatched at her overnight bag, dragging her off her feet while she clung and clung, the paving stripping skin from knuckles and elbows. A cluster of other ancients had gathered then and she was being helped up, her bag with its broken strap still at her feet.
>
> (Astley 1995: 145–6)

Awareness of vulnerability in later life can be triggered off by an unexpected street event when, for example, someone is suddenly the victim of a violent attack. One dark evening after finishing her meal at one of her favourite restaurants in London, Fanny Pye in Nina Bawden's *Family Money* walks out into a well-lighted residential area and witnesses a violent altercation between two motorists. One of the men is on the ground and when she intervenes to prevent his further harm she is knocked unconscious. Fanny is hospitalized for a short time and although she is not seriously damaged physically the attack triggers off a series of significant personal and social repercussions. Immediately following the attack Fanny's daughter Isobel visits her in hospital and is shocked to discover her mother has apparently rapidly aged. She seems to have been transformed from a 'strong, tall, supple woman, who had never to their knowledge spent a day in bed' to one who is now old. Her external appearance has apparently undergone a rapid transformation and she now looks much older, partly because she is bedridden and no longer conscious, and in her changed hospitalized condition she looks 'so vulnerable' (1997: 25).

Fanny herself also realizes that the physical attack has changed her personality. In a sense it has aged her prematurely in two ways: physically and mentally, influencing the subsequent decisions she makes about the course of her life. Psychologically she believes she is becoming forgetful and she worries about venturing onto the streets. She also begins, as previously noted, to feel that her children and friends may be conspiring against her to treat her as a child. She overhears a phone conversation between her cleaner Ivy and her son Harry where Ivy observes that she's 'a bit rambly' (1997: 54). Back home in bed, her mind restlessly ranges around the word 'rambly': 'Rambling, poor old thing, stubborn. Of course, you have to make allowances, she's had a nasty shock, but she's always liked her own way, you can't deny there's a selfish streak in her' (1997: 54).

Family risks

Bawden's *Family Money* offers a composite perspective on ageing from the viewpoints of Fanny as she experiences the attack and its consequences (physical, psychological and social) and her children whose concern about her welfare is complicated by their anxiety to persuade her to sell the family house so they can enjoy some of the profit. A story of ageing with these complex interpersonal dimensions helps to illuminate some of the intergenerational tensions, conflicts and contradictions that give ageing its peculiarly ambiguous quality. Readers can take in-depth account of the two sides of the story: the concerns of the children over their inheritance complicated by their genuine fears that after the attack Fanny may no longer be able to enjoy her previously fully independent life; and Fanny's subjective experience of physical injury and her struggle back to physical and mental stability. Much of the story is about how Fanny resists what she regards as efforts to infantilize her and regains her former self. In effect she rejects the vision of her future as an aged woman. During the course of her recuperation she thinks back to the attitude of her mother as she grew older:

> She must cling on to a sane way of thinking. People often became suspicious when they were ill. It was helplessness that brought it about. She had seen it happen to her mother when she grew deaf. She had complained that everyone muttered! She began to imagine they were all talking against her. . . . Although now, in her own case, it was natural that they should all be concerned. That didn't mean they had suddenly turned into enemies. Not her dear, loving children. Not Ivy, her friend!
>
> (Bawden 1997: 54–5)

As a story of ageing, *Family Money* displays some of the processes of interaction and the forms of conversation between members of different generations through which ageing is socially constructed (see Chapter 3). The unexpected physical attack which exposes the vulnerability of Fanny's body results in a sequence of interpersonal reactions which put her independent selfhood at risk and turn her life into a struggle to resist the efforts of her family to transform her condition into one of aged dependency. The attitudes of her children, well-intentioned as they like to think they are, threaten Fanny with transformation into an infantilized self. At the centre of this social interaction is a shift in the balance of power operating in the relationship of Fanny with her children. Infantilization threatens an older person's power of self-determination (Hockey and James 1993), and in her darkest hour Fanny is well aware of the precarious nature of her situation:

> There was always a point when the roles of parent and child were reversed; when the children took over. She must make it clear to them that in spite of her silly forgetfulness she had not reached that point yet. She was still in control of her own life; what she must do was to make decisions about her own future before they started to do it for her; take firm hold of the reins, stay one jump ahead. As soon as she felt a little less tired she would buckle down to it.
>
> (Bawden 1997: 55)

In this passage Fanny is opting for the self who, in the present, is suffering from a temporary physical illness but who can, once cured, return to the 'normal' self of the past. The distinction here is between illness as a curable affliction and the conception of ageing as an irreversible state of decline. In her imagination she is therefore rejecting the future of the aged self predicted by her children and she resolves to be her 'old' past self again and not allow her children to decide her future. Three of Fanny's selves are thus displayed in this narrative: the 'old' self of the immediate past, the physically ill self of the present, and the possibility of two selves in the future: an unwanted aged self or a return to the 'old' past self. Of course, the past 'old' self can never be replicated, but will be lived out in the light of recent events and changing circumstances.

Violation of the privacy of an older person is sanctioned when he or she is perceived as constituting a risk either to the self or others. Fanny Pye suddenly begins to suspect her children and helpers are uniting against her in what they regard as a benevolent conspiracy and she begins to fear this will lead to her loss of independence. The novelist Eva Figes likens this experience to that of becoming a kind of living ghost. The narrator of her poetic story of ageing, *Ghosts*, is an older woman whose house is being sold and her possessions dispersed. Serving tea to her son, his wife, and her daughter who are engrossed in dividing up her furniture and in a discussion of its use and value, she sees herself as 'a ghost on the periphery, watching. I am the child shut out. Overhearing, I want to join in. For now I am oblivious of the fact that it is not my turn. I have had my turn. It does not actually occur to me to live other than I do' (1989: 137).

In the form of a stream of consciousness, *Ghosts* invites us to see events through the older woman's eyes. But what is important is that she does not feel she has lost her youth. Although she feels herself to be a kind of insubstantial witness to events over which she has little control, she is also able to see things from her children's point of view and she can adopt the perspective of the other. Her private experience of ageing is essentially an interplay of the imagined perspectives of both youth and age: 'I have to see myself through their eyes to comprehend, through their eyes I see the chasm. I think back to my former self in order to forgive . . . I potter about in the kitchen, filling the teapot with hot water, unmissed, I think, hearing the voices rising and falling in the other room' (1989: 137–8).

Not every older person can forgive his or her relegation to the margins of life implied in the dispersal of the home, especially when it involves involuntary removal into residential accommodation. As we saw in some of the examples quoted in Chapter 4, a deep sense of anger rather than gentle resignation may be provoked, especially when an older person feels betrayed. Such a sense of betrayal is sharply realized in Thea Astley's *Coda*, when Kathleen, the central character, returns to her home to find that her daughter Shamrock has moved out all the furniture. The place is a 'void':

> Total. Tables, chairs, buffet had left only footprints on the linoleum. In the kitchen the space where the refrigerator had stood gaped its grimy outline. The stove had been wrenched from its cupboard fittings like an old tooth. Along the skirting board a cockroach moved disconsolately.
>
> (Astley 1995: 132)

When her daughter Shamrock appears at the empty house shortly after Kathleen has made her shocking discovery, she tells her mother that she has booked her into 'the most wonderful place' (p. 134): a retirement village called Passing Downs. Her house has been sold as part of a development from which Shamrock and her husband, Len, will profit. Kathleen is also told that the pair have had Brutus, her dog, put down:

> 'Oh God.' Kathleen wept hopelessly. Her eyes and nose streamed and she wiped carelessly at her melting face with the sleeve of her worn jacket. 'Oh God. I don't want to leave. I don't want to.'
> 'You've got no choice, Mum.'
> 'Don't Mum me, Shamrock. You've got the empathy of a piranha.'
>
> (Astley 1995: 136)

Not surprisingly, given the strong negative emotions that loss of independence can provoke, the fear of the physical and mental frailty associated with ageing is a common theme in fiction as in life. Mary Wesley's lively and thoroughly determined character Matilda Poliport, recently widowed, describes to a younger man she has met how she and her husband Tom anticipated ageing:

> 'We decided when we were still in our prime not to allow ourselves to crumble into old age where you are dependent on others, your powers fail, you repeat yourself, you become incontinent. The children try their best, then put you into an old people's home with nothing to look forward to but the geriatric ward. That is what we both minded about age, the keeping alive of useless old people. He and Louise [Matilda's daughter] used to have a game: how many children could eat if old people were allowed to die? Millions.'
>
> (Wesley 1991: 70)

Matilda's response is one others have considered – a determination to avoid the risk of a dependent future by committing suicide.

The risks of physical and mental frailty are very often anticipated threats to the ability to maintain an independent self. To borrow again from Leder (1990), with the extended life course there is always the possibility that processes of physical ageing and the illnesses associated with later life will dysappear and intrude on the experience of the self. Robert Barnard's crime story *At Death's Door* opens with an atmospheric description of the physical and mental decline of Roderick Cotterel who in his prime has been a controversial author and formidable hell-raiser. His body no longer silently interacts with his tempestuous personality and has finally let him down. Upstairs in his bedroom he is making a rambling effort to dictate his will into a tape-recorder; he pauses for a quarter of an hour after the effort:

> A dribble of saliva came from the corner of the old man's mouth and coursed down his chin. Eventually the forehead wrinkled, as if pale shadows of thought were going round in his mind. At last there was some movement under the bedclothes and slowly a hand emerged from under the sheets – a hand so little fleshed as to resemble a talon. Wavering, it felt its way to the little bedside table, and pressed down the switch on the portable tape-recorder that always sat there. The voice resumed, with a slight access of strength and determination.
>
> (Barnard 1990: 5)

Downstairs, Cotterel's family feel that his obsessive will-making is at least a sign of mental activity and preferable to the days 'when he's entirely passive' (1990: 6). Cotterel's decline has left him a burden not only to himself but to his immediate caregiving family. His immediate dependency grows into a threat to the entire stability of the family when figures from his colourful earlier life appear on the scene with potentially harmful secrets about his past. In one respect rather similar to Nina Bawden's *Family Money*, this story shows that older people themselves are not the only ones who are vulnerable to the risks of ageing. While the process of physical ageing has deprived Cotterel in person of his ability to behave badly and embarrass others, the written secret record of his past misdemeanours has empowered other people to cause considerable trouble in his name. Cotterel's decline has produced a shift in the balance of power to discomfort others; Cotterel's past self can no longer be activated in his own body but may be restored to harmful life through the actions of others. In this respect the story is an account of the unfolding of a series of social consequences following on from Cotterel's physical decline.

The manipulation and exploitation of infirmity

The idea that older people may easily be exploited through the manipulation of physical and mental infirmity provides a dramatic story-line for authors of crime fiction. In the words of Agatha Christie's Tuppence Beresford (*By The Pricking of My Thumbs*), if you wanted to put away a talkative elderly relative who might put you at risk by revealing a family secret you'd look for:

> A nice respectable Home for Elderly Ladies. You'd pay a visit to it, calling yourself Mrs Johnson or Mrs Robinson – or you would get some unsuspecting third party to make arrangements – You'd fix the financial arrangements through a firm of reliable solicitors. You've already hinted, perhaps, that your elderly relative has fancies and mild delusions sometimes – so do a good many of the other old ladies – Nobody will think it odd – if she cackles on about poisoned milk, or dead children . . . nobody will really listen. They'll just think it's old Mrs So-and-So having her fancies again – nobody will take any *notice at all*.
>
> (Christie 1994a: 49)

The work of Celia Dale is particularly interesting in this respect. In *Sheep's Clothing*, Grace and Janice first meet in Holloway Prison and get together to prey on older women pensioners who they believe keep valuables in their houses. They obtain access to private property by posing as officials of the DHSS (Department of Health and Social Security) who are concerned that the residents are not enjoying their full entitlement to benefit. A gender issue comes into play in this confidence trick. Grace and Janice prefer their victims to be women because they believe that men are less likely to have anything of value, their rooms are often disgusting and they are more likely to be suspicious and become difficult or attempt sexual molestation – 'even an old man could be surprisingly strong' (1990a: 26). Their technique is to lull their victim into a false state of security, get invited into the house, sympathetically engage her in conversation, induce her to make a cup of tea, drug the tea and steal her valuables. The 'beauty of the scheme' for Grace is the power to profit from the stereotypical weaknesses of older women: loneliness, respect for authority, physical and mental frailty; and the tendency of the police, operating with yet another stereotype of older women, to be sceptical about any complaints they might subsequently make:

> Like as not, the old dears didn't even know they'd been robbed for quite a time after her visit, and even then they probably thought they'd mislaid whatever it was, forgotten where they'd put it. And even when (and if) they did realise what had been done, they were too confused and ashamed to tell anyone. For if an old lady comes into a police station, agitated and probably deaf, and says she can't find her hubby's watch and chain that she's sure she always kept in a shoe-box at the back of the wardrobe but hadn't actually set eyes on since she couldn't remember when, what sort of tale is that?
>
> (Dale 1990a: 27)

Celia Dale draws on the stereotype of a specific kind of woman pensioner to create an engrossing story of ageing, but she also goes one step further by showing how misleading stereotypes of vulnerability can be. There is scope for error and miscalculation because not all older women are what they seem. Grace and Janice are seriously misled by the street appearance of Miss Andrews, lamed by arthritis. On closer inspection she becomes a force to be reckoned with: 'squat, with a square leathery face and a crop of white hair cut like a man's'. Grace 'instantly realised that, although she was lame and had walked with a stick all the way when Grace had trailed her from the Post Office, she was not frail' (p. 30). Miss Andrews lives up to Grace's reassessment of her character. She refuses to allow them into her kitchen to make a cup of tea, rejects the suggestion that she is disabled, contemptuously dismisses the prospect of benefiting further from 'charity', and in an abrupt manner forces them to leave her house.

Miss Andrews is sufficiently self-possessed to reject the category into which the conspirators wish to place her – 'dear' – and is consequently labelled 'an old cow' who 'could turn nasty' (p. 33). She is a threat to the conspirators because she doesn't comply with their assumption that older women pensioners are usually passive victims who don't ask questions or have very high expectations. As the story shows, there is a danger in stereotyping both to the older people on the receiving end and also to those who attempt to apply the labels.

But older people who are physically dependent in some way *can* be worn down no matter how resilient they may appear to be. In the same story, Celia Dale also shows how an older domineering woman can be progressively disempowered by a younger one who is absolutely determined to undermine her in the pursuit of personal advantage. Grace meets Conroy Robinson, a single man, whose mother is housebound with ulcerated legs and high blood pressure. She is the egotistical former actress, Marion Conroy, and until Grace intrudes into her domestic space she has Robinson at her beck and call. Ever the confidence trickster, Grace sets out to worm her way into Marion's confidence, eventually engineering a fall by greasing the bathroom floor with soap. Marion is now even more physically dependent and Robinson needs even more help with his mother, thus opening the way for Grace, posing as an expert in the care of older people, to move right into the house and take over. Celia Dale allows the reader to see how Grace is able to create a situation where Robinson is totally unaware of the way she is systematically reducing his mother to an increasingly dependent old age. She manipulates her relationship with Robinson and his mother by playing a dual role: solicitous about his mother to Robinson's face but humiliating his mother's physical dependence behind his back. In effect she transforms Marion into a stereotypical old woman who becomes afraid to complain to her son about her mistreatment:

> Her complaints sounded trivial, she knew. She could not bring herself to tell the more humiliating incidents, the roughness, the disregard of privacy, the wounding truths, for these would reveal her loss of power, the seeping away into the morass of old age of that dominance by which she had ruled her life and the lives of those near her. She could not admit, least of all to the son she had always commanded, that she was no longer supreme.
>
> (Dale 1990a: 159)

A new pattern of interdependencies has emerged. Robinson's domestic dependence on Grace makes him unwilling to give any credibility to his mother's knowledge that Grace is a 'wicked woman' (p. 169).

In this story Celia Dale provides us with what amounts to an interactionist perspective on one kind of risk to which older people may be exposed. We see exactly how Marion Conroy is manoeuvred into a position of extreme vulnerability and why it is possible for her son to be unwilling to believe her version of the process. We also see how it is possible for an exploitative character like Grace to manipulate an ageist stereotype.

Celia Dale provides another example of the manipulation of interactional skills to exploit an older person in *A Helping Hand*. Josh and Maisie Evans are a predatory middle-aged couple who first meet Mrs Cynthia Fingal, a lonely widow in her seventies, on holiday in Italy. Mrs Fingal has financial assets and Josh has well-developed social skills which he proceeds to deploy in order to establish a preliminary rapport when he takes her out to a café where:

> under his smiling attention she began to sparkle. She raised her chin as though to lift it clear of the dewlaps, stretched her neck as though it were still the column of creamy flesh on which the head, chestnut dark then, white now, used to ride so gracefully, sending slanting glances that had once ravished. From inside this heap of old flesh peeped a girl, a bride, a young mother, ridiculous and sad. Only half-listening to what she said, Josh registered her flowering. His kind eyes answered hers, although his thoughts were on the three German girls writing postcards at a nearby table, their thighs like copper beneath their shorts . . .
>
> (Dale 1990b: 22–3)

Attracted by the apparent sympathy and concern of Josh and Maisie, Mrs Fingal is seduced into leaving her niece, Lena, with whom she is reluctantly staying, to set up home in the spare bedroom of the Evans' bungalow. But just as a positive identity can flourish in the context of encouraging interaction with others, so it can be discouraged, reduced and destroyed. Once she has been lured into the bungalow the couple set out to weaken the links between Mrs Fingal and her niece, gradually depriving her of external support and making her more dependent on them. In effect she is gradually infantilized and the stereotype of childishness in old age is manipulated by Maisie to widen the gap between Cynthia and Lena and to reduce sympathetic communication between them even further. Josh and Maisie's aim, of course, is to persuade Cynthia to disinherit Lena in their favour. As Maisie says to Lena in the course of trying to make her believe her aunt thinks she is only interested in her inheritance, ' "Old people are very sweet but they do sometimes like to make things awkward, don't they, like children they are sometimes" ' (p. 84).

Celia Dale exposes the processes of social interaction through which an older person may be manipulated into dependency. From the beginning readers are fully aware of the malevolent motives of Josh and Maisie Evans but we are also given access to Mrs Fingal's subjective world; her distressing subjective experience of socially constructed dependence on Josh and Maisie so that she ultimately becomes a powerless witness of the conspiracy around her. Her vulnerability is compounded by the fact that appearances can often be misleading. The friendly Christian names 'Josh' and 'Maisie' conceal a calculating and hard-hearted exploitation of weakness and their bungalow is not a cosy and dependable haven of peace and safety, but in reality a kind of hellish prison for the luckless Mrs Fingal where her ageing is relentlessly accelerated.

In fiction residential care is not always displayed at its best, partly because the negative aspects of institutional care add a strong dramatic element (especially to a crime story) or are used as a narrative device, as we have seen, for stimulating strong emotion and 'human interest'. The image of residential accommodation as a place where the dependency of older people is deliberately contrived has been drawn on by a number of writers including Cath Staincliffe in *Go Not Gently*, where the main character is private investigator Sal Kilkenny. Sal is consulted by Agnes Donlan, an older woman concerned about the rapid decline she has seen in her friend Lily after she has been admitted into Homelea Nursing Home following a fall. Lily is no longer her usual self and is becoming more and more mentally frail and Agnes has been told that Alzheimer's disease is responsible for her friend's condition but she does not believe this explanation. Her question is: why did Lily change so rapidly from a normal socially competent person into an unresponsive nonperson: ' "I'm concerned," ' says Agnes, ' "that Lily's health is being affected, that something in that place is making her ill" ' (Staincliffe 1998: 2). When Sal accompanies Agnes on a visit to see her friend, Lily stares 'blankly, unwavering, at Agnes for two or three seconds' and then looks 'back to the television set'. It is clear to Sal that Lily does not recognize her friend and, after further deterioration, she is transferred to a psycho-geriatric unit. Again Agnes wants to know why the hurry? She does not believe that Lily is suffering from Alzheimer's disease but Sal remains unconvinced.

The interest in this story lies in the problematic nature of Alzheimer's disease and other dementias and the assumptions concerning their effects. Sal is faced with the task of testing out the validity of Agnes' belief that her friend is not really suffering from dementia and she goes to great lengths to consult the opinions of experts before taking her investigation further. A third of the way through the story she watches a TV documentary on abuse in private residential accommodation and keeps on seeing the faces of Agnes and Lily on the screen:

> What would Agnes do now? She'd been so certain that something was awry and we'd found nothing. She had to face the inevitability of her friend's illness and eventual death, though she could go on for years. In the books I'd read there were examples of people who had lost all sense of who they were, who no longer recognised family or friends, who'd lost all personality and needed constant care and reassurance. It would be hard for Lily but it'd probably be harder for Agnes to watch her friend disappear.

> (Staincliffe 1998: 63)

In the examples we have discussed so far, older people and their immediate friends and relations are perceived primarily as *victims of* the ageing process in two ways. First, the body dys-appears: internal biological changes affect physical and mental functions and make it more difficult for an older person to perform as a fully competent social self. These difficulties may be temporary or permanent in duration but in either case they have some effect on the inner and the outer self. Second, changes in physical and mental competencies can be exploited by other people for their own ends and their negative actions and communications can hasten the ageing process and deprive older people of their rights as fully social beings. In both cases older people may well appear in a pathetic light but this is only part of the story. As we saw in Stanley Middleton's *Live and Learn*, older people like the formidable Mr Hookes, who is aggressively armed against potential physical attack, can turn the tables.

Older characters as risk takers

Not all older fictional characters are described as passive victims – a stereotype that lures us into thinking that older people are more sinned against than sinning – and it is certainly misleading to think of old age as inherently virtuous. Indeed, there has always been a tendency, certainly in the Christian tradition, to make a moral distinction between virtuous old age as a preparation for Heaven and vicious old age as the forging ground of Hell. In this respect old age has never been seen as morally neutral although the grounds for moral distinction may be changing (Hepworth 1995a). The negative stereotype of the old witch is one obvious example of the capacity of the human imagination to attribute evil intent to older women. Witches, like the images of old bawds and procuresses who prey on young women and lure them into prostitution, have for centuries been seen as the epitome of what Simon Schama has described as 'wrinkles of vice and wrinkles of virtue'

(1988: 430). For men one negative stereotype is the 'dirty old man', a figure who still looms large in the popular imagination.

On the virtuous side, older people may be represented as exemplary risk takers. And they are not always described as physically frail. Simon Brett's Mrs Pargeter, a widow in her late sixties, is always exposing herself to danger in order to confront a criminal or solve a mystery, and she is by no means defenceless because she has on call the services of a devoted band of her deceased husband's criminal associates. Mrs Pargeter is a wealthy hedonist; a hearty individual who regards life as 'an unrivalled cellarful of opportunity to be relished to the last drop' (Brett 1990: 17), and she revels in her wealth (the results of her late husband's highly successful life of crime in which she did not participate). In *Mrs Pargeter's Package* the following description of her appearance is an explicit display of her wholehearted enjoyment of life:

> imperceptibly on the move from voluptuousness to stoutness. The golden hair, which, in an earlier existence . . . had turned many heads, was now uniformly white, but the clear skin, which had also been the subject of much compliment, still glowed with health. The backs of Mrs Pargeter's hands bore the tea-stain freckles of age, but her rounded legs, beneath their grey silk stockings, remained unmarked by veins. Mrs Pargeter, it could not be denied, was a very well-preserved lady.
>
> (Brett 1992a: 10)

For those fictional detectives who are less robust, physical frailty is usually portrayed as a kind of mask of ageing concealing superior mental powers and organizational skills. A good example occurs in Marianne Macdonald's *Death's Autograph*. Barnabus, a retired academic and heart attack victim who is supposed to take it easy at all times, uses his extensive experience of wartime intelligence to solve a murder mystery. Barnabus is the father of the central character Dido Hoare, and she worries constantly about the risks to his health:

> My father – seventy-two years old, widowed for five years, seven years retired from university teaching, and four months past his heart attack. For the last hundred and twenty days, I'd been afraid of losing him after all. Nowadays, when my telephone rings, I answer it – wet or dry, sober or drunk.
>
> (Macdonald 1996: 10)

The most popular risk-taking amateur detective to deploy the stereotype of the passively vulnerable old lady with a fuddled mental life is Agatha Christie's Miss Marple. She is the archetypal genteel English spinster whose most notable contribution to stories of ageing is the fact that she wears the *mask* of ageing (Light 1991; Shaw and Vanacker 1991; Hepworth 1993). Masking in this case refers to the mask as concealing rather than revealing inner character and Miss Marple's everyday appearance, as described by Anne Hart in *The Life and Times of Miss Jane Marple*, is highly deceptive as befits someone familiar with the darker side of humanity:

> Her hair was usually described as white, occasionally grey, her face as pink and crinkled, and her teeth as ladylike. She was tall and thin and

had very pretty china-blue eyes, which could look innocent or shrewd depending on one's point of view. Her general expression was usually described as sweet . . . but this could change when she was on the trail of someone evil.

(Hart 1991: 73–4)

Miss Marple is not exempt from some of the troubles of the dys-appearing body of later life – rheumatism, stiffening joints, and attacks of bronchitis and pneumonia – and she has had the occasional fall, but her mind is that of the steely-minded criminal investigator with a heightened awareness of the deceptive nature of the appearance of normality in the external world and a cool eye for the evil that lies beneath the surface of everyday life.

As we saw in Chapter 2, great value is placed in western culture on the eyes as expressive of an inner self in an ageing face, and Miss Marple is no exception to this rule. Not only does her expression change when contemplating a mystery, but her eyes shine 'very brightly, unusually so, considering her age' (Christie 1994b: 92). The contrast between the innocuous nature of her appearance and the triviality of her stereotypically spinsterish life is, say Shaw and Vanacker, the secret of her success and the key to her role as 'a powerful force for good'(1991: 63). This secret is, moreover, regarded as a cultural bridge between the world of fiction and assumptions about the role of older women in everyday life:

> The abilities old ladies possess – knowing what, how, and why something happened, and what ought to have happened – amount to the essential qualities of the detective: a strong moral sense, a knowledge of human nature, and a capacity for deduction based on carefully observed evidence. It is the 'trivial' lives of old ladies, who have plenty of leisure, the wisdom of experience, long memories, little personal drama in their own lives, and a huge capacity for vicarious living through observation of and gossip about the lives of others, that makes them into potentially excellent detectives.
>
> (Shaw and Vanacker 1991: 63)

And as Giles and Gwenda, the young couple with a mystery to solve in Christie's *Sleeping Murder* observe, no one is surprised when old ladies poke about asking questions: ' "It's quite a natural thing to do – for an old lady. . . . It's not as noticeable as though we did it" ' (1994b: 135).

Agatha Christie also draws on the contrast between physical frailty and mental ability in her story about the final days of her Belgian detective Hercule Poirot to which she gave the appropriate title *Curtain*.

Poirot, one of crime fiction's most popular private detectives, summons his former comrade Captain Hastings from Argentina to Styles Court in Essex. Styles Court, a large country house, was the scene of Poirot's first successful case and Christie's first successful novel in 1921. But it is now several decades later and Styles, in keeping with the broader pattern of social change, is no longer a private house but a private guest house where Poirot is now resident. On his journey to Styles, Hastings recalls his sense of shock and sadness at the changed appearance of his friend a year ago. Poirot 'was now a very old man, and almost crippled with arthritis' (Christie 1990: 6). On his arrival at Styles, Hastings is even more shocked at his first sight of Poirot and describes for readers the effects of 'the devastation wrought by age':

> Crippled with arthritis, he propelled himself about in a wheeled chair. His once plump frame had fallen in. He was a thin little man now. His face was lined and wrinkled. His moustache and hair, it is true, were still of a jet black colour, but candidly, though I would not for the world have hurt his feelings by saying so to him, this was a mistake. There had been a time when I had been surprised to learn that the blackness of Poirot's hair came out of a bottle. But now the theatricality was apparent and merely created the impression that he wore a wig and had adorned his upper lip to amuse the children!
>
> (Christie 1990: 14)

Poirot is, as he himself admits, a physical 'wreck', confined to his wheelchair and scarcely able to look after his physical requirements. But the point of the story, of course, is that he has not lost his masterly touch: '"Mercifully"', he says, '"though the outside decays, the core is still sound"' (1990: 15). And, as Christie's readers have come to expect, he is firmly in control of his final investigation; the processes of bodily ageing do not prevent him from bringing the murderer to justice. Poirot's brain continues to function with unimpaired accuracy.

In crime stories where older characters take risks their physical weaknesses are more than compensated by their intellectual ability to restore the moral balance in society. Moreover, they are interesting in terms of the situations in which they are found. The meanings symbolically ascribed to old age, as we have noted, are partly derived from the situations or social contexts of later life. And the situations provide the grounds for the social categorization and marginalization of age. Thus we *expect* to see older people in a geriatric ward and not in a youth club. Miss Marple is 'in place' when pictured in her cottage in the village of St Mary Mead, and also in place as a guest in the old-fashioned Bartram's Hotel in London. Poirot is in place as the invalid resident of a genteel private guest house. But at the same time these older characters are *out of place*; they put criminals at risk because they go against the grain of social stereotypes. As figures of the imagination they show how it is possible for us to be misled by the external appearance of older people and their apparent congruity with their physical surroundings. In terms of the age categorization process, these older characters perform their conventional social functions, but on another level they make us aware that age categorization contains some profoundly misleading constructs.

Death and control in old age

The fact that death is increasingly delayed until old age and indeed is now closely associated with the final period in the ageing process – 'dying on time' – results from our efforts to control both ageing and death in contemporary society. A number of strategies for exercising control in the face of prospective dying and death arise and are described in fiction. One technique involves efforts to exercise control over people long after one has died. Writers of wills, for example, realize that ageing need not necessarily mean loss of power over those who expect to benefit. Dorothy Rowe, the psychologist, has noted that the:

> traditional way of fighting back is to make a will. Then, whenever one of your possible beneficiaries seems likely to displease you, you can threaten to cut them out of your will. If the beneficiary persists in this wicked behaviour you can demonstrate that you have indeed done so.
>
> (Rowe 1994: 75)

In Nina Bawden's *Family Money*, Fanny, whose children believe her to be in the early stages of dependency and are anxious for her to sell her large house in London, wonders:

> if she were getting like Great-Aunt Frances who had died the year she was born. According to Fanny's mother, this old maiden aunt had kept a Black Book in which she wrote down her bequests to her nephews and nieces, making adjustments when they pleased or displeased her, or as the fancy took her. . . . Aunt Frances, apparently, had nothing much to give, a little jewellery, a nice porcelain tea set, three or four decent pieces of furniture. Her property, all the same, and to give or withhold it, was privilege and power.
>
> (Bawden 1997: 155)

Revenge for the actions of family members in the past is the grim theme of Francois Mauriac's *The Knot of Vipers* where the central character, Louis, a successful man aged 68, pours out in a letter to his wife his resentment of and desire to disinherit his family over the wrongs he believes he has experienced: 'It may be that I shall exert greater power over you when I am dead than I ever did while living . . .' (1985: 20). He is suffering from heart disease and is dying secretly in his country house in Calese in the vine region of Bordeaux in France:

> It is exactly as though a hand were gripping my left shoulder and keeping it rigid in a strained position, so that I may never be allowed to forget, for a moment, what's lying in wait for me. In my case, death certainly won't come by stealth. It has been snuffing around me for years. I can hear it and feel its breath. It treats me with patience because I make no effort to resist, because I submit to the discipline which its approach imposes. I am ending my life in a dressing-gown, surrounded by all the paraphernalia of incurable disease, sunk in the great winged chair where my mother sat waiting for her end.
>
> (Mauriac 1985: 18)

In Alison Lurie's *The Last Resort* the main character, a 'world famous writer and naturalist' Wilkie Walker, who is aged 70, and his younger wife Jenny, aged 46, have gone to Key West for a vacation where Wilkie will complete his latest book on the species of tree called the copper beech. But he has come to believe that he is dying of cancer and, unwilling to disclose his fear to Jenny, he sits in his study all day pretending to write his last book. In reality he is spending his days planning his 'accidental' death by drowning at sea.

Wilkie's unwillingness to discuss his worries with his wife leads to deep misunderstandings all round and a breakdown in communication. Jenny, misled by Wilkie's secrecy concludes that his coolness towards her is because he is having an affair, and he comes to believe the same of her. Later, when Wilkie undergoes what he thinks is a heart attack, and is discovered in the ensuing medical examination in hospital not to have cancer, he finds that he has been transformed from the man who at the beginning of the novel was described as having aged well to one who looks much older. He is therefore not seriously ill but is physically altered and on one of her visits to the hospital Jenny observes the extent of his transformation:

> It wasn't like him to apologize, to worry about his health. It was like another person. And as she thought this, Wilkie began to change while she watched, from a strong, handsome, healthy, but cold and unfaithful husband into a heavy, slack, elderly person with gray chenille hair and irrational fears.
>
> (Lurie 1999: 227–9)

Wilkie also is conscious of himself as old, but he is also aware that now he is not really ill at all he will have to carry on writing, giving lectures, 'playing the worn-out part of Wilkie Walker, formerly famous naturalist and environmentalist' (p. 229). In other words, he must now play the role of the scholarly elder statesman with at least the consoling thought that he may enjoy renewed popularity among an older audience who have the resources and time to attend his lectures in luxury surroundings.

In Mauriac's *The Knot of Vipers*, the letter and disclosure of Louis' plan of revenge is a comment on years of distorted communication in a loveless marriage; on the deep resentment of Louis, who in the end comes to terms with his life and moves, in his letter-writing to a form of repentance. The letter is in the end a confession: a life-review from the perspective of one man's inner self on his own life. Louis acts in anticipation of his death in the belief that some time still remains to complete his long letter. Although seriously ill, he still has time to look back on his life and recall his grievances.

The violent death of an older person is interesting in crime fiction partly because it may arise out of some well-kept secret from the past, and this allows an investigation of individual motives and convoluted personal relationships. Secrets, as we saw in Chapter 3, play a highly significant role in interpersonal relationships. In Agatha Christie's *Hercule Poirot's Christmas* the murder victim is Simeon Lee of Gorston Hall, a man who made his fortune through wheeling and dealing in South Africa when he was young. He has had a checkered past and, now old, brings his family together for Christmas, seemingly to torment and goad them and to enjoy their discomfort and embarrassment – a Christmas to remember. Lee, an unpleasant man, has not been mellowed by old age but retains his power to control and taunt his family through his enormous wealth. Christie's description of Lee gives a striking contrast between his physical ageing and the appearance of an invalid, and the impression of wealth and power, and the mental energy which makes it possible for him to continue to scheme and plot. There is also an intimation of malevolence in the reference to the 'clawlike' hands:

In a big grandfather armchair, the biggest and most imposing of all the chairs, sat the thin, shrivelled figure of an old man. His long clawlike hands rested on the arms of the chair. A gold-mounted stick was by his side. He wore an old shabby blue dressing-gown. On his feet were carpet slippers. His hair was white and the skin of his face was yellow.

A shabby, insignificant figure, one might have thought. But the nose, aquiline and proud, and the eyes, dark and intensely alive, might cause an observer to alter his opinion. Here was fire and life and vigour.

(Christie 1993: 33)

The occurrence of violent death offers the novelist an opportunity to explore the negative aspects of human relationships and the continuing influence of the past on the present and into the future. In Marianne Macdonald's murder mystery *Ghost Walk*, Dido Hoare, an antiquarian bookseller, finds an unconscious old man in her doorway. She recognizes him as an occasional customer, Tom Ashe, who appears to be down and out, aged 'seventy or older, but it's hard to tell with the homeless: they don't wear well' (1997: 4). Essentially the mystery turns around the identity of Ashe who is eventually murdered and who has mysteriously made Dido the executor of his estate. Solving the mystery of his identity resolves the motive and the identity of the murderer.

Another problem associated with old age which serves to intensify the mystery is the question of Ashe's state of mind. His way of life and actions seem puzzling. He lived in an abandoned factory when he had over £30,000 in his bank account. His wife, who is suffering from cancer lives in a nursing home in Brighton and appears to talk in riddles. A letter Ashe leaves behind is so cryptic that it could have been written by someone who has become senile.

Murder and the subsequent disentanglement of the secret pertain to interesting questions of human motivation. Because the secret is the motive it raises the question of the identity of the murder victim. What was she or he like? What had he or she done in the past to warrant such a violent end? Ann Granger's crime story *A Word After Dying* opens with the sudden death of Olivia Smeaton, a recluse living in the large 250-year-old Rookery House in the Cotswold village of Parsloe St John. She is described as physically frail though mentally robust, steely and resolute. An independent person with whom no one wishes to tangle. She also has the advantage of living in an old, large and delapidated house, has had a colourful past and comes from a wealthy family. (The delapidation is not surprising: see the discussion in Chapter 4 on affinities between people and places.) Although the bare factual details of her past life are known, and described briefly in her obituary in the local newspaper, no one has any idea why 'her final years were spent in near seclusion' (1997: 31). And then there is the question of a motive for investigating a person's past.

This casts an interesting light on old age because old people in such stories are portrayed as a sort of unknown. In a sense they are personified solely as older persons with no known past and a comparatively short-term future. It is the people who investigate the crime who must construct the victim's life course by formulating a convincing narrative of the connections between past, present and future. The writer of imaginative fiction is free to make these connections, to fill in the details of a lifelong process of ageing within the covers of a book. The murder of a frail old person is thus the first stage in dramatizing a motive which is often located buried deep in the past. And the dramatization of the motive requires the dramatization of the life course: the symbolic interplay noted by Mead between past, present and future.

One powerful source of dramatic narrative and also one with significant everyday implications is the possibility that the threatening or dangerous behaviour of an older character may originate in the physical/mental abuse to which they were exposed in the past. This is a notable theme in Minette Walters' *The Scold's Bridle*. The investigation of the grotesque murder of an upper-class older woman, Mathilda Gillespie, in her bathroom at Cedar House reveals a background of sexual abuse and exploitation by the male members of her family. Suffering from arthritis and embittered towards men, she keeps a diary recording the secret history of her family life and her harsh judgements on human relationships. Proud and arrogant with a 'vicious tongue' (1995: 26) she reveals a convoluted and embittered pattern of family relationships which include sexual deviation and blackmail. Her diaries are her revenge and excerpts from them form an interweaving theme throughout the novel. She also leaves behind her a 'video will' describing her rape by her uncle at the age of 13, and the hostility of her father to whom she revealed her sexual exploitation 12 years later. He put the blame for his brother's conduct on her, calling her 'a disgusting slut' and declining 'to do anything' (p. 76). She goes on to record her eventual resort to blackmail and her disillusionment with her daughter and granddaughter, bequeathing a considerable amount of the money they had expected to inherit to someone outside the family – her doctor. The investigation into her murder, during the course of which excerpts from the diaries are gradually revealed, opens up Mathilda's family history and explains why she has become a dangerous old woman and why someone decided to ensure her silence.

Mathilda is a vengeful old woman who, we discover, is as much sinned against as sinning. The tangle of relationships in her exploitative family distorts an individual with talent and potential that results ultimately in a vicious crime. Mathilda's power is a morally perverted power. To some extent she can be described in later life as displaying the 'wrinkles of vice'.

Another example of a dangerous older woman, the malignity of whose complex personality has been shaped from childhood, can be found in Lesley Glaister's *The Private Parts of Women*. Inis, a wife with a young family, runs away from her doctor husband and comfortable home in a bid for freedom in 'a dreary little house in a dreary post-industrial city' (1996: 1). Her next-door neighbour in this run-down area is Trixie Bell, aged 84, at first sight an ordinary rather drab old woman living in equally drab surroundings: 'an ordinary old woman, wandering a bit perhaps, but that's normal surely at her age' (p. 52). But the story unfolds to admit the reader behind the commonplace façade of Trixie's backstreet existence, for she, rather like Max Montfalcon in Hope's *Serenity House*, inhabits a nightmarish subjective world. Gradually Inis discovers that Trixie is not simply a salvationist whose energetic hymn-singing can sometimes be heard through the wall at night, but a person with three distinctive selves – and one of these multiple selves is very dangerous indeed. Trixie's house is not simply the 'shell of the self' but the shell of *selves*, and as we read the novel she is transformed from a simple confused old woman into a serious threat to Inis' liberty and life.

6

Futures

All the stories of ageing we have looked at in this book are structured according to the conventions of a narrative form in which time flows in a linear fashion from the past through the present to the future. It is normally the case, writes Dorothy Rowe, that 'all proper stories' have 'a beginning, a middle, and an end': the beginning is 'where we come from', the middle is 'the present time' and the future is 'the working out of our story'. Our sense of self 'evolves with the sense of time passing, and our life story is an essential part of our sense of self' (Rowe 1994: 47). Any narrative, writes Margaret Gullette, implicitly 'tells a story of life-over-time' (1997: 86).

Past, present and future

In our stories of ageing time is seen as linear, moving inexorably from the past to the future and shaping the human life course into a series of 'ages' and 'stages'. The model of the human life span divided into 'ages' or 'stages' has a long history which continues to influence our imaginings and expectations of the ageing process (Hepworth 1995b). In, for example, Marika Cobbold's *A Rival Creation* Evelyn Brooke, the older character who is an expert horticulturist and ardent promoter of nature conservancy, typically compares her own human life course with that of a tree in the natural world: ' "You're just resting," she murmured, running her hand down the rough bark of the copper beech that spread its naked branches across the top lawn. "But for me it's terminal. Autumn leads to winter, but there will be no spring. Your life is a circle, mine is a line. Lucky you" ' (1994: 86).

In this traditional model, human life change is seen as following a pattern prescribed by nature. According to this interpretation it is perhaps not surprising that older people should be stereotyped as resistant to change. The old gardener in Agatha Christie's *Sleeping Murder* contemptuously compares the unwelcome 'changes' of urban life with stability of country life: a predictable regularity of the seasons; an unchanging pattern of planting for renewed growth (1994b: 18–19).

Yet in one sense ageing in western culture has always been oriented towards the future and such an orientation inevitably implies change. Death, the biggest change of all in western mainstream religious thought, has never been the end of the story. And whether we subscribe to religious ideas or not in present-day society, the dualistic belief in the separation of the body from the soul still persists in the difficulty all of us experience in imagining the end of self. This is reflected, for example, in attempts to influence events after one has died by leaving behind a sardonic suicide note or a last will and testament giving those left behind a piece of one's mind (Louis' letter to his wife in Mauriac's *The Knot of Vipers*) or a 'video will' passing judgement on others for their shortcomings (Mathilda Gillespie's vindictive video-will in Walters' *The Scold's Bridle*). There is more than a suspicion, too, that the author of a deliberately unsettling last will and testament may somehow continue to enjoy the discomfort of those who have been disinherited. An indication, perhaps, of the capacity for interaction to persist after death in the symbolic realm.

The potential of the self to persist after death is also recognized, as we have seen in Chapter 4, in the belief in ghostly hauntings and in the idea that past lives may in some way impregnate the fabric of material places and possessions. As Jenny Hockey has suggested, the central symbolic role of the home in the experience of the self is expressed in the haunted house where the present occupants of a property experience an invasion by 'the hidden selves of others' (1999b: 160). The 'hidden selves of others' are former occupants who have in some way been closely identified with the house. The anxiety, fear and anger that surround haunted houses can be partly attributed to the close association between place and selfhood which symbolically transcends time. Haunted houses and haunted families justify the belief in the persistence of the self beyond the material world into a form of immortality (Finucane 1982). Ghosts and hauntings symbolically express the wish of humans to influence others when they are out-of-body and out-of-life, and ageing in this view is not the end of the self or the story of the self, though it may well induce the body to dys-appear.

It is, of course difficult to estimate how many people still believe in the power of supernatural forces to intrude into everyday life in the material world, but there seems to be little doubt that many of us believe in the persistence of the self after death. As Leder (1990) argued, our ability to ignore the physical body which is the basis of our existence – to treat it for much of the time as if it is absent when we are free from pain and dysfunction – encourages us to believe that the self can exist in some disembodied way. And, as I have argued in this book, the role of symbols in social life – their power to free us from the natural world from which we have evolved (Elias 1991) – provides considerable scope for a belief in the extension of the self beyond its material frame. The power of the human imagination, saturated as it is in symbolic forms, enables us to enjoy the experience of 'living on' in the homes, personal possessions, images and memories we leave behind. Thus we all, potentially at least, experience an ageless self. And because the self is a social product deriving from and dependent upon interaction with other human beings we can glean some assurance of the continuity of personal identity through the promised support of family, friends and carers. Research clearly shows that even when the memory has apparently been incapacitated by dementia, the self can be kept socially alive through the caring efforts of others (Kitwood 1998; Sabat 1998). The self becomes a group treasure, safeguarded and passed almost ritually from one carer to another. For Linda Grant, after living through her mother's confusion and ultimate admission into residential care, the future of ageing is ultimately memory, for memory 'is everything, it's life itself' (1998: 17); and when those who remember us have gone we may persist symbolically solely in the documents we have left behind: 'we will exist, one day, only on paper and writing will be all that's left of us' (Grant 1998: 37).

As we have noted on several occasions, our awareness of the problematic nature of the future is sharpened by our reflexive personal observations of the ways those around us age and eventually die. In Penelope Lively's *Passing On*, the death of Edward Glover's mother makes him aware of time passing, of his own ageing, and the limitations of his own future: 'Nothing lasts, he wept, everything goes. My mother is dead, who had always been there, for better and for worse. Mostly for worse. And I am forty-nine and getting old and soon it will be too late for all the things I know nothing of but which will torment me in the middle of the night' (1989: 57).

One of the issues we have to face increasingly as we grow chronologically older arises out of Mead's observation that human action is always oriented towards an imagined future. The 'I' is experienced as fleetingly suspended in the present between reflections on the past and the future. And the realization that we have moved away from the past at a more rapid rate than we imagined can sometimes come as an unsettling surprise. Jane, the middle-aged heroine of Nicci French's *The Memory Game*, looks back on the apparent speed with which her children have grown up and left her behind:

> They practise being grown-up for such a long time, and then one day you notice that they really are grown-up. Where had all that time gone? How had it happened that I was middle-aged and on my own, and never again would I know the swamping joy of holding a child under my chin and saying: Don't fret, it'll be all right, I promise you it'll be all right.
>
> (French 1998: 225)

The shifting balance between time lived and time left to live, recorded in Jane's reflexive awareness that her children have 'grown up' and Edward Glover's reaction to the death of his mother, brings us face to face with the question of anticipatory ageing: what will it be like to be old in the future? And as Gullette (1997) has forcefully reminded us, the process of biological ageing raises questions about social attitudes towards the future of ageing which are particularly pressing in a youth-oriented culture where older people are relentlessly relegated to the margins of social life. One response to the ageing question is to attempt to extend the margins of middle age as far into the imagined future as is possible in an effort to stifle or repress the thought that we shall ever grow old. This process requires us to distance ourselves from our own ageing by distancing ourselves from associations with any groups categorized as 'old'.

At the end of Simon Brett's *A Nice Class of Corpse*, Mrs Pargeter, at the age of 67 decides she will leave the Devereux private hotel on the south coast which caters for genteel, active retired people:

> She looked around at the other residents, and she realised again what they all had in common. They didn't look forward; they looked backwards. They had all finished their lives. They had all come to the Devereux to spiral down to a genteel death.
>
> And that was where the late Mr Pargeter's widow differed from them. She still had a lot to look forward to.
>
> No, she thought, as she rose from her armchair and went to tell Miss Naismith she would be leaving the Devereux, I'm not finished yet.
>
> (Brett 1992b: 186–7)

In Alison Lurie's novel *The Last Resort*, Lee, a middle-aged woman, ruminates over the conventional popular view that growing older means running out of time: 'Lee remembered something she had read once, that as you grow older and the future shrinks, you have only two choices: you can live in the fading past, or, like children do, in the bright full present' (1999: 253).

Personal attitudes towards the experience of time passing, and the relative values attached to past, present and future, vary from individual to individual. Studies of reminiscence work show there are wide differences in attitudes towards memories of the past (some people, for example, prefer to spend their later lives immersed nostalgically in the past while others are preoccupied solely with the present, and there are those who live vigorously towards the future), but there is no dispute over the vital role of reminiscence in maintaining a sense of continuity, personal identity and self-worth (Coleman 1993). One of the problems is that in order to engage in this process of personally constructing the meaning of ageing one must be in control of one's cognitive faculties, particularly memory. Working memory is unfortunately not always under our conscious control and the individual capacity to control reminiscence and access to one's inner subjective world can, as we know, be tragically undermined by dementia. Writing of a photograph of her mother, showing a confident, young woman posed with an arm resting on the bow-fronted window of her neat suburban villa, Linda Grant says:

> When she stood in front of the camera that day so long ago, she could confidently guess what the years to come would hold: prosperity; motherhood, the satisfaction of her own home. Now she has no sense at all of the progress of her memory's ebb. I do. She does not know what lies ahead and I'm not going to tell her.
>
> Soon, she will no longer recognise me, her own daughter. . . .
>
> (Grant 1998: 17)

The idea of human motivation as essentially oriented towards the future works well as long as our mental processes are unimpaired and as long as there is some kind of acceptable future to imagine. Until socially and personally acceptable forms of human life can be prolonged into the indefinite future most of us will have to come to terms with a lengthening past, the fleeting present, and a shrinking future. For some of us this restricted future will most certainly include exposure to the risk of mental confusion and some form of intrusion into the routine social life of the dys-appearing body. Even when life may be prolonged through bio-medical interventions (as is frequently predicted for the twenty-first century), millions of the earth's inhabitants will be excluded from its immediate benefits.

Coming to terms with the future as a finite resource will for some be seen as an act of 'surrender' to time, conceived as an enemy, as in the following description of a man in his fifties from Simon Williams' *Talking Oscars*: 'It was an honest, healthy face whose features were elegantly surrendering to his fifty-odd years. Deep lines furrowed his dark skin and wings of grey hair swept back from his temples . . .' (1989: 20). For others, as the research of Gullette (1997), Jerrome (1993), Williams (1990) and others shows, it will be a prolonged effort to age positively and resist decline. For yet others it will be a challenge to our survivalist sense of humour, a view expressed by the novelist Kingsley Amis during an interview about the television version of his black comedy on ageing *Ending Up*. While, he said, 'nobody can make old age and pain bearable, you can make the thought of it bearable. At least one can laugh about it – till it arrives' (Furness 1989/90: 21).

The future of ageing is therefore highly ambiguous and it is not surprising that images of the past, or the past as remembered, and its influence on the immediate present have tended to play a more central role in stories of ageing than speculations about the future. As we have seen, even master detectives like Hercule Poirot eventually come to their last case and Miss Marple does become frailer, though both continue to find their razor-sharp intellects unimpaired. One interesting feature of stories about the influence of memories of past events is the way memory is described as an essentially fluid process with a capacity to deceive at any 'age' or 'stage' of life. A good example of the tricks memory can play and the resulting mental confusion in those who are not suffering from any form of dementia can be found in Nicci French's *The Memory Game*, in which the discovery of the body of a young woman who disappeared several years ago forces her now middle-aged friend Jane to seek therapy and eventually to become aware that her memory of the past has been highly misleading. She has, in other words, been living for much of her life with an illusion. Such a discovery can, of course, exercise a dramatic influence over the personal experience of ageing.

While fiction does tend to work with the conventions of narrative time it is also, as the product of the creative imagination, freer than empirical social gerontology to manipulate conventional sequences of time and memory. Pat Barker's Geordie in *Another World* is, at the age of 101, haunted by his traumatic experiences in the trenches during the First World War. He does not believe he is dying from cancer but that his death is the long-delayed result of a bayonet wound received in battle all those years ago. Barker uses this vision of the influence of the past to open up an alternative view of time as a circular process where the past, present and future continuously interrelate. Time ceases to be linear but fuses in essence with the present and prospectively with possible futures. In this sense Geordie believes he is being killed by the past which cannot be reduced to merely a haunting memory.

James Long's novel *Ferney*, about reincarnation, is another (and as a work of fiction quite different) example of the way writers can deconstruct the linear concept of time and offer an alternative vision of the future of ageing. Ferney, an old man in appearance, is a reincarnated form of life who has witnessed centuries of historical events and is thereby an integral feature of the history of the physical environment.

Science, technology and the ageing body

For centuries in western culture ageing has been imagined as a condition of existence from which human beings can only be rescued by supernatural forces. True, there has always been the quest to prolong active life, but until very recently the search has been a dream rather than a reality. And when people have experienced eternal life it has more often than not been a curse rather than a blessing, as in the legends of The Wandering Jew and The Flying Dutchman. Sometimes supernatural forces do intervene in the apparently natural order of things to arrest the normal processes of physical ageing, as happens in the case of Faust (Fiedler 1986), who makes a pact with the Devil and sells his own soul, and in Oscar Wilde's novel about moral corruption *The Picture of Dorian Gray*. Dorian Gray is an aesthete with wondrous good looks whose face and body remain mysteriously unmarked by his excessive indulgence in immoral practices; all external signs of his debauchery (in this story a form of premature ageing) are mysteriously transferred to his portrait. When he finally attacks the painting with a knife in an attempt to destroy the evidence of his past he succeeds only in destroying himself, so close has the affinity between the portrait and himself become. On his death the portrait reverts back to the original image of youth – 'all the wonder of his exquisite youth and beauty' (1960: 167) – leaving his dead body unrecognizably that of an old man, 'withered, wrinkled, and loathsome of visage' (p. 167).

Outside the realms of legend and the romantic imagination there was until very recently only one future of ageing in western culture if one was lucky to live long enough to grow older: the Christian vision of the inevitable decline of the human body, death and an afterlife of either Heaven or Hell. The dualistic separation of the body from the soul in Christian thought regards the ageing of the body in the temporal world as a brief testing ground for eternal spiritual life beyond the veil. The corruption of the flesh frees the soul or essential self for an other-worldly existence out of time. Heaven is the compensation for graceful or virtuous ageing and not looking for pacts with the Devil to prolong a youthfully active life.

But times are rapidly changing and the emergence of modern scientific medicine and technology has offered an alternative promise of release from the ageing of the body in this world rather than the next (Katz 1996). One of the interesting features of this development is that contemporary models of an ageless future have become predominantly biological rather than essentially spiritual (Cole 1992). The prevailing belief now is that it is the science of the biological body, and not the religion of the eternal immaterial soul, which will arrest the processes of ageing and extend the period of youthful life. The prominent social gerontologist Jaber F. Gubrium (1986) has commented on our reluctance in contemporary society to accept the 'normality' of a biologically limited life span. The widespread faith in the limitless potential of science to solve human problems encourages us to turn expectantly to medical science to transform ageing from the natural termination of the life course into a disease which is potentially curable. In this optimistic vision of the future of ageing the biological risks associated with later life will be curable and the human life span extended well beyond the biblical threescore years and ten. One of these days ageing will disappear from the human agenda when cures for the illnesses associated with growing older have been found and ailing and malfunctioning body parts can be replaced.

One way of defeating the ageing process is for humans to become cyborgs or to assume the 'post-human' bodies of partly biological and partly technological beings (Featherstone 1995). To return again to Leder's (1990) concept of the dys-appearing body, this vision of the future is one where the dys-appearing body literally *disappears*. Any part of the internal body which causes distress in later life will be removed and replaced with a genetically engineered or transplanted substitute. The story of the ageing body will thus become not a story of how individuals cope or come to terms with its limitations but science fiction come true. The body will be a machine and the meaning of ageing may cease to be a matter of concern.

For some analysts the future of ageing lies in cyberspace, the electronically constructed environment where reality is 'virtual', and life is a 'post-human utopia'. In cyberspace we don't replace our ageing bodies or turn ourselves into cyborgs to halt the wear and tear but simply leave the body behind as we embrace the disembodied experience. In cyberspace, bodies are not the point at which human interpersonal interaction begins but are replaced by flexible and manipulable images of bodies. Cyberspace offers the attractive prospect of liberation from the body especially if we feel our bodies are unattractive or are letting us down in some way. The limitations of the ageing body in everyday social life are left behind and symbolic liberation enters a new dimension of experience. In this futuristic scenario of ageing, human beings have the potential of becoming transformed into disembodied, electronic, cyber-selves.

Futures of ageing

Raymond Tallis (1999: 23) has argued that 'the debate on the implications of the ageing population is highly negative. Gloomy about the present and doomy about the future'. Negative factors include mounting pressures on the health services and an unequal balance between the numbers of producers and later-life dependants. But he also argues an alternative and more optimistic vision of the future. While ageing may remind us of the physical limits to existence, it also provides the opportunity for 'a new kind of life beyond the traditional, largely unchosen narratives of ambition, development and personal advancement; and the biological imperatives of survival, reproduction and child-rearing' (1999: 230). In other words, a new kind of story. But what kind of story of the future of ageing can be written?

There are a number of stories which either use ageing as a vehicle for exploring the future or incorporate images of ageing into a futuristic scenario. In his Introduction to the 1977 edition of the *The Poorhouse Fair* John Updike describes his novel, about the older people who are living in an American state-run institution, the Poor Home, as a 'vision of the future' (1990: ix). The novel was written in 1957 and set 20 years into the future but there is in this vision no end to old age as presently understood. The old in the Poor Home are by no means futuristic creatures – times may change but ageing does not. Much more recently Updike has written in *Toward The End of Time* about the theme of the ageing body and its relation to the self in the context of a novel set in the year 2020. He projects his story of time as a limited resource, in an image of an America which has been ravaged and therefore radically changed by a Sino-American War. The Midwest is devastated, cities such as Boston have been drastically reduced and organized society has fragmented, leaving the maintenance of law and order to a system of private contract where only the wealthy can pay for the security of their property. Ben Turnbull is a retired broker in his sixties and subject to the same physical changes and concerns with the male self that can be found in novels about ageing in contemporary society. Like countless other men before him, Turnbull gazes into the shaving mirror and sees the same kind of changes: 'the wreck of the flesh – the eyelids so sagging their folds snag one another and need to be rubbed back into place upon waking, the double cords of throat wattle, taut only when I lift my chin to shave beneath it . . .' (1999: 51). The descriptions of his experience of his body, internal and external, are graphically similar in terms of their preoccupations with other novels which are not set in the future.

Although Updike's novel is set in the future it is not the biological, personal and social aspects of ageing which have changed, but the infrastructure of society. The preoccupations of the ageing male with which we are familiar in the present – sexual potency, anxiety over the meaning of life etc. – remain unchanged in this vision of the twenty-first century. For Updike the biological processes of ageing are an inescapable characteristic of the natural world unfolding within the natural 'flux' of the universe (1999: xvi).

As far as stories of ageing are concerned, futures can be imagined in two different ways. First, in terms of radical cultural change, and second in terms of the extreme bio-technical restructuring of the internal and external body outlined above. For cultural critics like Gullette (1997) the future should be seen as presenting an opportunity to reject the several centuries of ageism which have been responsible for stories of ageing as decline in favour of a new type of age identity which refuses to associate physical changes in later life with any form of diminution of individual competence to make a full contribution to society. In other words, in the cultural change scenario of the future ageing is given a value in its own right. Efforts are not made to disguise the signs of ageing or to restructure biology, but rather to gain acceptance for the idea that ageing is a period in the life course of potential self-realization and social growth.

One way of combating ageism is to consider the potential for a cultural reconstruction of the life course. Critics are now arguing, especially from a post-modern perspective, that culture is becoming more diverse, the life course is becoming more complex, and the traditional 'ages and stages' of life model is fragmenting and becoming more fluid. As a consequence the self is becoming more complex. Individuals are losing their identification with a grounded locality and relatively stable set of social relationships and consequently are becoming more diverse in later life. This is reflected in the increasingly complex personal archive. Many people in the past had only tiny collections of photographs, personal mementos, letters and records of their past life. The exception was the aristocracy with its large houses full of portraits, and more recently photographs, and attics full of records. Stella Tillyard's (1995) book about the four Lennox sisters between the years 1744–1832 is based upon such a collection. A rich family archive where the vicissitudes of the life course are closely traced in correspondence between daughters of the rich and well-connected family of the second Duke of Richmond. Tillyard writes of the 'astonishing richness of my sources – thousands of letters, pictures, household accounts and rules, an inventory, library lists, travel journals, prayers, verses, autopsies, maps, parks and buildings' (p. xi) which allowed her to construct a picture of the life histories from childhood into old age of Emily, Louisa, and Sarah. And in this work, which includes interesting descriptions of the experiences of illness and ageing, Tillyard sets out to remind us of the similarity and differences between their lives and our own.

But for most ordinary people the fact remains that such records were never kept or only existed in miniaturized replicas in the boxes under the bed and the cases in the attic we have seen in some of the stories of ageing discussed in previous chapters. In my own family, many of the old photographs were kept in a large cardboard box secured with rubber bands. I have now inherited the cardboard box containing the family photographs I used to study closely and our musty and cumbersome late Victorian photograph album containing images of family members (several unknown) in their best clothes. This small collection stands in contrast to the drawers of photographs and videos that represent the record of my own generation's life. And I well remember the time and effort we put into weeding out the photographs and slides we wanted to keep after my father died. As our own images accumulate so does the record of potentially multiple selves over a lifetime. But the diversity of selves and identities that will be open to us as we age is still an open question and one that only experience will prove.

Glenda Laws (1995) saw the promise of an 'emancipatory perspective' in the post-modern landscapes, as she describes them, of Sun City in the USA. If we remember that an important source of the concept of post-modernity is architecture then it is fitting that these retirement communities – landscapes within which people age – may be seen as sites of the post-modern fluidity of age identity. The reorganization of the spatiality of ageing is seen as highly significant. These 'new, [post-]modern spatial arrangements are central to the redefinition of ageing and the aged' (Laws 1995: 275). This is because they foster images of the body as actively retired, thus eroding the traditional fixed or appointed places for ageing – the hearth of the Victorian granny, the rocking chair – and requiring the ability to move around, to pick and choose, to experiment, to recreate the self and experiment with new identities. An example of the cultivation of independent living away from the family home can be found in Francine Stock's character Daphne in her novel *A Foreign Country*. Although her husband is still alive and has suffered a stroke, Daphne lives alone in the seaside cottage that was once the family holiday home. Here she cultivates her own lifestyle and maintains contact with her husband. Here is no image of a Darby and Joan but that of a formidable woman who has done demanding intellectual and professional work and is thoroughly able to age positively on her own terms.

Two last questions

Mead saw that the structure and nature of the external social order exercises a profound influence over everyday human relationships and the quality of self-consciousness. Changes in the social organization of society produce changes in patterns of social interaction which in turn influence the self or selves, or roles that individuals can take. Because symbolic interactionism is about the interdependence of body, self and society it does not envisage a fixed status quo but continuous change. I have suggested throughout this book that symbolic interactionism offers a valuable perspective on ageing because of its emphasis on change as the continuous and inescapable condition of social life. From this perspective the more complex our society the more possibility there is for developing multiple selves in response to a widening network of human associations, and ultimately for expanding the range of stories about ageing. Kitwood's (1998) positive approach to persons suffering from Alzheimer's disease is a specific example of how ideas of the self as a social construct open up the possibility of socially preserving the individuality and dignity of someone who is ill.

Ultimately, as Wilkie Walker in Alison Lurie's *The Last Resort* rather ironically observes, older people are the future. And, in Christopher Hope's *Serenity House*, the owner Cledwyn Fox describes the 'guests' of his 'eventide Home' as 'us':

> 'Do you know who they are, Mr and Mrs Turberville? The guests of Serenity House? I shall tell you. They're *us*! That's who they are. If we're lucky. In a way I regard them as veterans from the wars of life. And sometimes as spacemen or deep-sea divers, out of their usual atmosphere. Out of their depth. Do you think they need our pity? God forbid. Do you know what they do need? Equipment! Explorers venturing into another age, having to cope in a totally new environment. Our elders are also innovators, Mrs Turberville. That's what they are. When I look at my guests, what do I feel for them? I'll tell you – gratitude. That's what I feel. Where they lead we will surely follow tomorrow.
>
> (Hope 1993: 50–1)

One way of handling the problematic nature of the past and the continuously shifting balance between the past and the future in later life is to try to turn experience into an endless present. In Sutton's *Gorleston*, Percy, now widowed and retired, reflects on the change in his experience of time since he was younger, when Saturday night had a special meaning in the working week:

> Now, so much later in Gorleston, there was no favoured evening to go out. There was no Saturday night or Friday night or Wednesday night. Every night was the same. Every night people went out, if they could, if they were mobile, to console themselves for some loss or other. In his timeless retirement Percy found that many things quickly assumed extraordinary dimensions and proportions, with scant regard for the past. . . . For in Gorleston people lived for the moment. The past was hazy. There was not much future.
>
> (Sutton 1995: 86)

The idea that ageing is the end of future – the point, as the joker puts it, when we run out of it – partly depends not on the chronological duration of the future we can expect to live but on a shift in emphasis in the quality of experience that is desired. At the very end of Barbara Pym's *Quartet in Autumn*, Letty, now retired, takes a much more optimistic view than Percy when she understands that 'life still held infinite possibilities for change' albeit, it is implied, in terms of the small-scale subtleties of everyday life (1994: 176). In other words, the possibilities of change are not located in anticipation of the length of time one has left to live but in a recognition of the human potential that exists in even the smallest details of everyday life. From this perspective an optimistic view of the future diverts attention away from the prospect of an extended future towards a concern with the richness of life on a much smaller scale. The changes may be tiny but they are nonetheless momentous.

Any consideration of the possible future of ageing inevitably takes us back to the central concern of this book: namely, the quality of the processes of symbolic interaction between body, self and society from which the experience of ageing is constructed. This, as we have seen, is a process open to movement and change and the future of ageing is therefore uncertain. We can close, therefore, with two important questions about the future of ageing. The first concerns each one of us as individuals and asks: how do we imagine our own future as ageing human beings? The second relates to the wider social context within which stories of ageing are written and asks: what is our cultural vision of the ageing process in the future? Do we imagine one unifying future of ageing or can we anticipate a variety of alternative futures of ageing? If so, how do they differ from what we know already, and what will they be like? They are, of course, the subject for another book.

There remains one final point. It seems to me that there is a real sense in which stories of ageing which eliminate the ageing body either through the invocation of divine or demonic forces or, more plausibly perhaps, through innovations in electronic communication and the promise of the cyborg, are not really stories of ageing at all. The stories of ageing we have explored in this book are, in one or another of their variations, about how individuals and groups make sense of biological change. What they do not do is to reduce ageing to a 'merely' bio-medical issue (simply a matter of the body), and they often dignify later life by imagining ageing as a struggle for personal meaning and social significance. If we all become 'ageless' cyborgs we are transformed into machines which, like any other, simply require regular servicing to keep on going to the end of the road. But the end of the road in this vision in an infinitely extending horizon leading who knows where. It seems to me that if the body does not age then there simply is no story of ageing to tell. Or to put the issue slightly differently, in the words of Kathleen Woodward: 'the grandiose fantasy of eliminating altogether the inevitable process and consequences of ageing reveals a prejudice against ageing that is harmful to all of us' (1999: 291).

References

Non-fiction

Bailin, M. (1994) *The Sickroom in Victorian Fiction: The Art of Being Ill*. Cambridge: Cambridge University Press.

Benson, J. (1997) *Prime Time: A History of the Middle Aged in Twentieth Century Britain*. London and New York: Longman.

Berger, A.A. (1997) *Narratives in Popular Culture, Media and Everyday Life*. London: Sage.

Blaikie, A. (1999) *Ageing and Popular Culture*. Cambridge: Cambridge University Press.

Blythe, R. (1981) *The View in Winter*. Harmondsworth: Penguin.

Bond, J. (1993) Living arrangements of elderly people, in J. Bond, P. Coleman and S. Peace (eds) *Ageing in Society: An Introduction to Social Gerontology*, 2nd edn. London: Sage.

Bond, J., Briggs, R. and Coleman, P. (1993) The study of ageing, in J. Bond, P. Coleman and S. Peace (eds) (1993) *Ageing in Society: An Introduction to Social Gerontology*, 2nd edn. London: Sage.

Burkitt, I. (1991) *Social Selves: Theories of the Social Formation of Personality*. London: Sage

Bytheway, B. (1985) *The Later Part of Life: A Study of the Concept of Old Age*, occasional paper no. 10. Swansea: School of Social Studies, University College of Swansea.

Bytheway, B. (1995) *Ageism*. Buckingham: Open University Press.

Chapkis, W. (1986) *Beauty Secrets: Women and the Politics of Appearance*. Boston, MA: South End Press.

Chappell, N.L. and Orbach, H.L. (1986) Socialization in old age: a meadian perspective, in V.W. Marshall (ed.) *Later Life: The Social Psychology of Ageing*. London: Sage.

Christie, A. (1978) *An Autobiography*. Glasgow: Fontana.

Cohen, A. (1994) *Self Consciousness: An Alternative Anthropology of Identity*. London: Routledge.

Cohen, G. (1987) Introduction: the economy, the family, and the life course, in G. Cohen (ed.) *Social Change and the Life Course*. London and New York: Tavistock.

Cole, T.R. (1992) *The Journey of Life: A Cultural History of Ageing in America*. Cambridge: Cambridge University Press.

Cole, T.R. and Winkler, M.G. (1994) *The Oxford Book of Ageing: Reflections on the Journey of Life*. Oxford: Oxford University Press.

Coleman, P. (1993) Adjustment in later life, in J. Bond, P. Coleman and S. Peace (eds) *Ageing in Society: An Introduction to Social Gerontology*, 2nd edn. London: Sage.

Corbin, A. (1986) *The Foul and the Fragrant: Odour and the French Social Imagination.* Leamington Spa: Berg.

Coupland, N., Coupland, J. and Giles, H. (1991) *Language, Society and the Elderly.* Oxford: Blackwell.

Crimmens, P. (1998) *Storymaking and Creative Groupwork with Older People.* London and Bristol, PA: Jessica Kingsley.

Csikszentmihalyi, M. and Rochberg-Halton, E. (1981) *The Meaning of Things: Symbols and the Self.* Cambridge: Cambridge University Press.

Daily Mail (1995) Together for ever, the old lady and a threadbare friend, 27 October: 25.

Davidoff, L. and Hall, C. (1987) *Family Fortunes: Men and Women of the English Middle Class 1780–1850.* London: Hitchinson.

Drabble, M. (1979) *A Writer's Britain: Landscape in Literature.* London: Thames & Hudson.

Elias, N. (1985) *The Loneliness of the Dying.* Oxford: Basil Blackwell.

Elias, N. (1991) *The Symbol Theory.* London: Sage.

Fairhurst, E. (1999) Fitting a quart into a pint pot: making space for older people in sheltered housing, in T. Chapman and J. Hockey (eds) *Ideal Homes? Social Change and Domestic Life.* London and New York: Routledge.

Featherstone, M. (1995) Post-bodies, ageing and virtual reality, in M. Featherstone and A.Wernick (eds) *Images of Ageing: Cultural Representations of Later Life.* London and New York: Routledge.

Featherstone, M. and Hepworth, M. (1993) Images of ageing, in J. Bond, P. Coleman and S. Peace (eds) *Ageing in Society: An Introduction to Social Gerontology*, 2nd edn. London: Sage.

Fiedler, L. (1986) More images of eros and old age: the damnation of Faust and the fountain of youth, in K. Woodward and M.M. Schwartz (eds) *Memory and Desire: Ageing – Literature – Psychoanalysis.* Bloomington, IN: Indiana University Press.

Finucane, R.C. (1982) *Appearances of the Dead: A Cultural History of Ghosts.* London: Junction Books.

Furness, A. (1989/90) The famous 5, *TV Times*: 21.

Goffman, E. (1968) *Stigma: Notes on the Management of Spoiled Identity.* Harmondsworth: Penguin.

Goffman, E. (1969) *The Presentation of Self in Everyday Life.* Harmondsworth: Penguin.

Grant, L. (1998) *Remind Me Who I Am, Again.* London: Granta Books.

Gubrium, J.F. (1986) *Oldtimers and Alzheimer's: The Descriptive Organisation of Senility.* Greenwich, CT: JAI Press.

Gubrium, J.F. (1995) *Individual Agency, the Ordinary and Postmodern Life.* Milton Keynes: School of Health and Social Welfare, Centre for Ageing and Biographical Studies, The Open University.

Gullette, M.M. (1988) *Safe at Last in the Middle Years: The Invention of the Midlife Progress Novel: Saul Bellow, Margaret Drabble, Anne Tyler, and John Updike.* Berkeley, CA: University of California Press.

Gullette, M.M. (1993) Creativity, ageing, gender: a study of their intersections, 1910–1935, in A.M. Wyatt-Brown and J. Rossen (eds) *Ageing and Gender in Literature: Studies in Creativity.* Charlottesville, VA and London: University Press of Virginia.

Gullette, M.M. (1997) *Declining to Decline: Cultural Combat and the Politics of the Midlife.* Charlottesville, VA and London: University Press of Virginia.

Hallam, E., Hockey, J. and Howarth, G. (1999) *Beyond the Body: Death and Social Identity.* London and New York: Routledge.

Hart, A. (1991) *The Life and Times of Miss Jane Marple.* London: Sphere.

Hepworth, M. (1993) Old age in crime fiction, in J. Johnson and R. Slater (eds) *Ageing and Later Life*. London: Sage.

Hepworth, M. (1995a) Wrinkles of vice and wrinkles of virtue: the moral interpretation of the ageing body, in C. Hummel and J. Lalive D'Epinay (eds) *Images of Ageing in Western Societies*. Geneva: University of Geneva, Centre For Interdisciplinary Gerontology.

Hepworth, M. (1995b) Change and crisis in mid-life, in B. Davey (ed.) *Birth to Old Age: Health in Transition*. Buckingham: Open University Press.

Hepworth, M. (1996) William and the old folks: notes on infantilization, *Ageing and Society*, 16: 423–41.

Hepworth, M. (1998) Ageing and the emotions, in G. Bendelow and S.J. Williams (eds) *Emotions in Social Life: Critical Themes and Contemporary Issues*. London and New York: Routledge.

Hepworth, M. (1999) In defiance of an ageing culture, *Ageing and Society*, 19: 139–48.

Hepworth, M. and Featherstone, M. (1974) 'Persons believed missing': a search for a sociological interpretation, in P. Rock and M. McIntosh (eds) *Deviance and Social Control*. London: Tavistock.

Hepworth, M. and Featherstone, M. (1982) *Surviving Middle Age*. Oxford: Basil Blackwell.

Hockey, J. (1999a) The ideal of home: domesticating the institutional space of old age and death, in T. Chapman and J. Hockey (eds) *Ideal Homes? Social Change and Domestic Life*. London and New York: Routledge.

Hockey, J. (1999b) Houses of doom, in T. Chapman and J. Hockey (eds) *Ideal Homes? Social Change and Domestic Life*. London and New York: Routledge.

Hockey, J. and James, A. (1993) *Growing Up and Growing Old: Ageing and Dependency in the Life Course*. London: Sage.

Hollander, A. (1988) *Seeing Through Clothes*. Harmondsworth: Penguin.

Hoskins, J. (1998) *Biographical Objects: How Things Tell the Stories of People's Lives*. New York and London: Routledge.

James, A. (1995) On being a child: the self, the group and the category, in A.P. Cohen and N. Rapport (eds) *Questions of Consciousness*. London and New York: Routledge.

Jay, M. (1994) *Downcast Eyes: The Denigration of Vision in Twentieth-Century French Thought*. Berkeley, CA: University of California Press.

Jerrome, D. (1992) *Good Company: An Anthropological Study of Old People in Groups*. Edinburgh: Edinburgh University Press.

Jerrome, D. (1993) Intimate relationships, in J. Bond, P. Coleman and S. Peace (eds) *Ageing in Society: An Introduction to Social Gerontology*, 2nd edn. London: Sage.

Johnson, J. and Slater, R. (eds) (1993) *Ageing and Later Life*. London: Sage.

Katz, S. (1996) *Disciplining Old Age: The Formation of Gerontological Knowledge*. Charlottesville, VA and London: University Press of Virginia.

Kaufman, S. (1986) *The Ageless Self: Sources of Meaning in Late Life*. Wisconsin, WI: The University of Wisconsin Press.

Kent, S. (1991) Introduction, in J. Cotier *Nudes in Budapest*. London: Aktok.

Kern, S. (1996) *Eyes of Love: The Gaze in English and French Painting and Novels 1840–1900*. London: Reaktion.

Kitwood, T. (1998) *Dementia Reconsidered: The Person Comes First*. Buckingham: Open University Press.

Laws, G. (1995) Embodiment and emplacement: identities, representation and landscape in Sun City retirement communities, *International Journal of Ageing and Human Development*, 40(4): 253–80.

Laws, G. (1997) Spatiality and age relations, in A. Jamieson, S. Harper and C. Victor (eds) *Critical Approaches to Ageing and Later Life*. Buckingham: Open University Press.

Lawton, J. (1998) Contemporary hospice care: the sequestration of the unbounded body and 'dirty dying', *Sociology of Health and Illness*, 20(2): 121–43.

Leder, D. (1990) *The Absent Body*. London: University of Chicago Press.

Light, A. (1991) *Forever England: Feminity, Literature and Conservatism Between the Wars*. London and New York: Routledge.

Lord, G. (1998) *James Herriot: The Life of a Country Vet*. London: Headline.

Lowenthal, D. (1986) *The Past is a Foreign Country*. Cambridge: Cambridge University Press.

Lyman, K.A. (1998) Living with Alzheimer's disease: the creation of meaning among persons with dementia, *The Journal of Clinical Ethics*, 9(1): 49–57.

Martin, B. (1990) The cultural construction of ageing: or how long can the summer wine really last? in M. Bury and J. Macnicol (eds) *Essays on Social Policy and Old Age*. Egham: Department of Social Policy and Social Science, Royal Holloway and Bedford New College (Social Policy Papers no. 3: 33–81).

Owen, B. (1995) *Summer Wine and Vintage Years: A Cluttered Life*. London: Robson.

Plummer, K. (1997) *Telling Sexual Stories: Power, Change and Social Worlds*. London and New York: Routledge.

Rooke, C. (1992) Old age in contemporary fiction: a new paradigm of hope, in T.R. Cole, D.D. Van Tassel and R. Kastenbaum (eds) *Handbook of the Humanities and Ageing*. New York: Springer Publishing Co.

Rowe, D. (1989) *The Construction of Life and Death*. London: Fontana.

Rowe, D. (1994) *Time on Our Side: Growing in Wisdom, Not Growing Old*. London: Harper-Collins.

Sabat, S. (1998) Voices of Alzheimer's disease sufferers: a call for treatment based on personhood, *The Journal of Clinical Ethics*, 9(1): 35–48.

Schama, S. (1988) *The Embarrassment of Riches: An Interpretation of Dutch Culture in The Golden Age*. London: Fontana.

Schwartz, H. (1989) The three-body problem and the end of the world, in M. Fehrer (ed.) *Fragments for a History of the Human Body, Part Two*. New York: Zone.

Shaw, M. and Vanacker, S. (1991) *Reflecting on Miss Marple*. London and New York: Routledge.

Stewart, A.G. (1977) *Unequal Lovers: A Study of Unequal Couples in Northern Art*. New York: Abaris Books.

Stuart, M. (1998) Writing the self and the social process, in C. Hunt and F. Sampson (eds) *The Self on the Page: Theory and Practice of Creative Writing in Personal Development*. London and Philadelphia, PA: Jessica Kingsley.

Tallis, R. (1999) Old faces, new lives, *The Times Higher*, 9 July.

Thompson, P., Itzin, C. and Abendstern, M. (1990) *I Don't Feel Old: The Experience of Later Life*. Oxford: Oxford University Press.

Tillyard, S. (1995) *Aristocrats: Caroline, Emily, Louisa and Sarah Lennox 1740–1832*. London: Vintage.

Turner, B.S. (1995) Ageing and identity: some reflections on the somatization of the self, in M. Featherstone and A. Wernick (eds) *Images of Ageing: Cultural Representations of Later Life*. London: Routledge.

Vaughan, D. (1988) *Uncoupling: How and Why Relationships Come Apart*. London: Methuen.

Williams, R. (1990) *A Protestant Legacy: Attitudes to Death and Illness Among Older Aberdonians*. Oxford: Clarendon Press.

Wood, L.A. (1981) Loneliness and life satisfaction amongst the rural elderly. Paper presented at the joint meeting of the Canadian Association on Gerontology and The Gerontological Society of America, Toronto, November.

Wood, L.A. (1988) Loneliness, in R. Harré (ed.) *The Social Construction of Emotions*. Oxford: Basil Blackwell.

Woodforde, J. (1983) *The Strange Story of False Teeth*. London: Routledge & Kegan Paul.

Woodward, K. (1980) *at last, The Real Distinguished Thing: The Late Poems of Eliot, Pound, Stevens, and Williams*. Columbus, OH: Ohio State University Press.

Woodward, K. (1991) *Ageing and its Discontents: Freud and Other Fictions*. Bloomington, IN and Indianapolis: Indiana University Press.

Woodward, K. (1999) From virtual cyborgs to biological time bombs: technocriticism and the material body, in J. Wolmark (ed.) *Cybersexualities: A Reader on Feminist Theory, Cyborgs and Cyberspace*. Edinburgh: Edinburgh University Press.

Wyatt-Brown, A.M. (1988) Late style in the novels of Barbara Pym and Penelope Mortimer, *The Gerontologist*, 28(6): 835–9.

Wyatt-Brown, A.M. (1992) *Barbara Pym: A Critical Biography*. Columbia and London: University of Missouri Press.

Ylanne-McEwen, V. (1999) 'Young at heart': discourses of age identity in travel agency interaction, *Ageing and Society*, 19: 417–40.

Zeilig, H. (1997) The uses of literature in the study of older people, in A. Jamieson, S. Harper and C. Victor (eds) *Critical Approaches to Ageing and Later Life*. Buckingham: Open University Press.

Fiction

Note: the dates of publication are those of the editions consulted and not necessarily the dates of first publication.

Amis, K. (1987) *Ending Up*. Harmondsworth: Penguin.

Amis, K. (1996) *The Biographer's Moustache*. London: Flamingo.

Astley, T. (1995) *Coda*. London: Secker & Warburg.

Bailey, P. (1987) *At The Jerusalem*. London: Penguin.

Barker, P. (1982) *Union Street*. London: Virago.

Barker, P. (1986) *The Century's Daughter*. London: Virago.

Barker, P. (1998) *Another World*. London: Viking.

Barnard, R. (1990) *At Death's Door*. London: Corgi.

Barnard, R. (1992) *Posthumous Papers*. London: Corgi.

Bawden, N. (1997) *Family Money*. London: Virago.

Braine, J. (1987) *These Golden Days*. London: Methuen.

Brett, S. (1990) *Mrs, Presumed Dead*. London: Pan.

Brett, S. (1992a) *Mrs Pargeter's Package*. London: Pan.

Brett, S. (1992b) *A Nice Class of Corpse*. London: Pan

Brookner, A. (1995) *A Private View*. London: Penguin.

Caveney, P. (1995) *Skin Flicks*. London: Headline.

Christie, A. (1985) *At Bartram's Hotel*. London: Fontana.

Christie, A. (1990) *Curtain: Poirot's Last Case*. London: Fontana.

Christie, A. (1993) *Hercule Poirot's Christmas*. London: HarperCollins.

Christie, A. (1994a) *By The Pricking of My Thumbs*. London: HarperCollins.

Christie, A. (1994b) *Sleeping Murder*. London: HarperCollins.

Clarke, R. (1987) *Gala Week*. Harmondsworth: Penguin.

Cobbold, M. (1993) *Guppies for Tea*. London: Black Swan.

Cobbold, M. (1994) *A Rival Creation*. London: Black Swan.

Conlon, K. (1986) *Face Values*. London: Coronet.

Cook, D. (1988) *Missing Persons*. London: Headline.

Dale, C. (1990a) *Sheep's Clothing*. London: Penguin.

Dale, C. (1990b) *A Helping Hand*. London: Penguin.

Dexter, C. (1990) *The Wench is Dead*. London: Pan.

Dickens, C. (1985) *Great Expectations*. Harmondsworth: Penguin.

Dibdin, M. (1994) *The Dying of the Light*. London: Faber & Faber.
Doughty, L. (1999) *Honey-Dew*. London: Scribner.
Ewing, B. (1997) *The Actresses*. London: Little, Brown & Co.
Figes, E. (1989) *Ghosts*. London: Flamingo.
Forster, M. (1978) *The Seduction of Mrs Pendlebury*. Harmondsworth: Penguin.
Forster, M. (1990) *Have the Men Had Enough?*. London: Penguin.
French, N. (1998) *The Memory Game*. London: Penguin.
Gilbert, A. (1987) *The Spinster's Secret*. London: Pandora.
Glaister, L. (1996) *The Private Parts of Women*. London: Bloomsbury.
Granger, A. (1991) *Say It With Poison*. London: Headline.
Granger, A. (1997) *A Word After Dying*. London: Headline.
Harvey, J. (1996) *Easy Meat*. London: Mandarin.
Hegarty, F. (1996) *Let's Dance*. London: Penguin.
Herriot, J. (1973) *If Only They Could Talk*. London: Pan.
Herriot, J. (1979) *All Things Wise and Wonderful*. London: Pan.
Hill, R. (1987) *Exit Lines*. London: Grafton.
Hill, R. (1993) *Recalled to Life*. London: Grafton.
Hill, R. (1999) *On Beulah Height*. London: HarperCollins.
Hill, S. (1999) *The Service of Clouds*. London: Vintage.
Hope, C. (1993) *Serenity House*. London: Picador.
Huth, A. (1998) *Land Girls*. London: Abacus.
Ignatieff, M. (1994) *Scar Tissue*. London: Vintage.
Isler, A. (1996) *The Prince of West End Avenue*. London: Vintage.
James, P.D. (1986) *A Taste for Death*. London: Faber & Faber.
Lee, L. (1962) *Cider With Rosie*. Harmondsworth: Penguin.
Lessing, D. (1996) *Love Again*. London: Flamingo.
Lively, P. (1983) *The Road to Lichfield*. London: Penguin.
Lively, P. (1989) *Passing On*. London: Andre Deutsch.
Lively, P. (1992) *City of the Mind*. London: Penguin.
Lively, P. (1998) *Spiderweb*. London: Viking.
Long, J. (1998) *Ferney*. London: HarperCollins.
Lurie, A. (1999) *The Last Resort*. London: Vintage.
Macdonald, M. (1996) *Death's Autograph*. London: Hodder & Stoughton.
Macdonald, M. (1997) *Ghost Walk*. London: New English Library.
Mauriac, F. (1985) *The Knot of Vipers*. London: Penguin.
Meade, C. (1989) *The Thoughts of Betty Spital*. London: Penguin.
Middleton, S. (1991) *Beginning to End*. London: Hutchinson.
Middleton, S. (1995) *Toward the Sea*. London: Hutchinson.
Middleton, S. (1996) *Live and Learn*. London: Hutchinson.
Middleton, S. (1997) *Brief Hours*. London: Hutchinson.
Middleton, S (1999) *Necessary Ends*. London: Hutchinson.
Moggach, D. (1989) *Driving in the Dark*. London: Penguin.
Moggach, D. (1997) *Close Relations*. London: Heinemann.
Newman, A. (1989) *A Sense of Guilt*. London: Penguin.
Pym, B. (1980) *A Few Green Leaves*. New York: E.P. Dutton.
Pym, B. (1994) *Quartet in Autumn*. London: Flamingo.
Rathbone, J. (1995) *Intimacy*. London: Victor Gollancz.
Rathbone, J. (1998) *Blame Hitler*. London: Indigo.
Rendell, R. (1995) *Simisola*. London: Arrow.
Renwick, D. (1992) *One Foot in The Grave*. London: Penguin.
Robinson, P. (1988) *Gallows View*. Harmondsworth: Penguin.
Rowntree, K. (1997) *Mr Brightly's Evening Off*. London: Doubleday.
Rubens, B. (1997) *The Waiting Game*. London: Little, Brown & Co.

Sackville-West, V. (1989) *All Passion Spent*. London: Virago.

Sarton, M. (1992) *As We Are Now*. London: The Women's Press.

Sarton, M. (1993) *Mrs Stevens Hears the Mermaids Singing*. London: The Women's Press.

Sherriff, R.C. (1974) *The Fortnight in September*. London: Arrow.

Smiley, J. (1995) *At Paradise Gate*. London: Flamingo.

Staincliffe, C. (1998) *Go Not Gently*. London: Headline.

Stock, F. (1999) *A Foreign Country*. London: Chatto & Windus.

Sutton, H. (1995) *Gorleston*. London: Sceptre.

Taylor, E. (1995) *A View of the Harbour*. London: Virago.

Taylor, E. (1996) *Mrs Palfrey at The Claremont*. London: Virago.

Trollope, J. (1993) *The Men and the Girls*. London: Black Swan.

Updike, J. (1990) *The Poorhouse Fair*. London: Penguin.

Updike, J. (1999) *Toward The End of Time*. London: Penguin.

Vine, B. (1996) *The Brimstone Wedding*. London: Penguin.

Walters, M. (1995) *The Scold's Bridle*. London: Pan.

Wesley, M. (1991) *Jumping the Queue*. London: Black Swan.

Wilde, O. (1960) *The Picture of Dorian Gray*, in G.F. Maine (ed.) *The Works Of Oscar Wilde*. London and Glasgow: Collins.

Williams, S. (1989) *Talking Oscars*. London: Mandarin.

Williams, S. (1993) *Kill the Lights*. London: Mandarin.

Index

UNDERSTANDING OLDER HOMELESS PEOPLE

Maureen Crane

This is a remarkable book, based on Maureen Crane's many years of acquaintance with homeless people. It throws light on the pathways which lead to homelessness, and should be required reading not only for policy makers in this field, but all those interested in the vicissitudes of the human life course.

Peter G. Coleman, Professor of Psychogerontology,
University of Southampton, UK

Drawing on 10 years experience of working with the elderly homeless, Maureen Crane has produced a book that will be of immense value to those who wish to understand more about this growing social problem.

Bryan Lipmann, Victoria, Australia

This book is destined to become the standard reference for anyone interested in ageing and homelessness.

Carl I. Cohen, Professor, Department of Psychiatry,
State University of New York Health Science Center at Brooklyn, USA

Although ageing people are a significant segment of the homeless population, they have largely been ignored by service providers and policy makers. This remarkable book sets out to remedy this situation and offers new research on the causes of homelessness. Partial life histories have been collected from older homeless people and their pathways into homelessness traced. Although the book is about older homeless people, many of them have been homeless since they were teenagers or since early adulthood. It therefore examines the reasons for homelessness at all stages of the life course. The book discusses the circumstances, problems and needs of older homeless people, looks at how services are responding, and makes recommendations for service development. Case studies are used throughout to assist explanations.

This book has much to offer a wide audience including service-providers, policymakers, healthcare workers, housing and social services workers, gerontologists and sociologists. Because it is easy to read, it is accessible to lay readers. It will be of interest to a British audience and an international audience, particularly in countries such as America and Australia where innovations in services for homeless older people are rapidly developing.

Contents

224pp   0 335 20186 5 (Paperback)   0 335 20187 3 (Hardback)

THE PSYCHOLOGY OF GROWING OLD
LOOKING FORWARD

Robert Slater

Readable and memorable. . . . If you have a particular interest in the psychology of ageing I recommend that you obtain a personal copy, as it is an up-to-date summary of present knowledge.

Nursing Times

A welcome contribution. . . . Slater demonstrates throughout his book a depth of reading and knowledge that is never less than impressive, enabling him to place the issues raised within a strong philosophical context that informs and broadens the issues.

Health Psychology Update

Captivating in its multi-disciplinary approach.

Ageing and Society

Ageing has traditionally been seen as ubiquitous decline – all 'doom and gloom'. *The Psychology of Growing Old* challenges this view and shows how our own attitudes and values may serve to perpetuate it. The book uses the research literature of gerontology – the multi-disciplinary study of ageing and later life – to involve the reader in considering his or her own future and that of others. It examines the potential that ageing and later life have to be a rewarding experience – something to look forward to – rather than something to be denied and rejected. Unlike other books in the area, *The Psychology of Growing Old* places the reader centre stage as someone who can influence the future of ageing. It will be of interest to a wide range of professionals in health and social services who work with older people; and relevant to many student courses with ageing as a focus, whether in psychology, sociology, nursing, gerontology, social work or the medical professions.

Contents
Introduction – 'Us' and 'them' – On being older – Coping and failing to cope – Speed of behaviour – Our changing brain – Belonging – Looking back – Finding meaning – Reconstruing reality – References – Index.

176pp   0 335 19318 8 (Paperback)   0 335 19319 6 (Hardback)

AGEISM

Bill Bytheway

Ageism has appeared in the media increasingly over the last twenty years.

- What is it?
- How are we affected?
- How does it relate to services for older people?

This book builds bridges between the wider age-conscious culture within which people live their lives and the world of the caring professions. In the first part, the literature on age prejudice and ageism is reviewed and set in a historical context. A wide range of settings in which ageism is clearly apparent are considered and then, in the third part, the author identifies a series of issues that are basic in determining a theory of ageism. The book is written in a style intended to engage the reader's active involvement: how does ageism relate to the beliefs the reader might have about older generations, the ageing process and personal fears of the future? To what extent is chronological age used in social control? The book discusses these issues not just in relation to discrimination against 'the elderly' but right across the life course.

The book:

- is referenced to readily available material such as newspapers and biographies
- includes case studies to ensure that it relates to familiar, everyday aspects of age
- includes illustrations – examples of ageism in advertising, etc.

Contents
Part 1: The origins of ageism – Introduction: too old at 58 – Ugly and useless: the history of age prejudice – Another form of bigotry: ageism gets on to the agenda – Part 2: Aspects of ageism – The government of old age: ageism and power – The imbecility of old age: the impact of language – Get your knickers off, granny: interpersonal relations – Is it essential?: ageism and organizations – Part 3: Rethinking ageism – Theories of age – No more 'elderly', no more old age – References – Index.

158pp   0 335 19175 4 (Paperback)

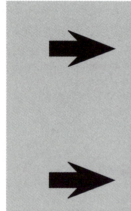